FEMINIST ETHICS AND SOCIAL POLICY

FEMINIST ETHICS AND SOCIAL POLICY
Towards a New Global Political Economy of Care

Edited by Rianne Mahon and Fiona Robinson

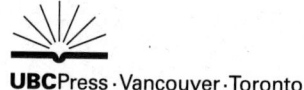

UBCPress · Vancouver · Toronto

© UBC Press 2011

All rights reserved. No part of this publication may be reproduced, stored in a retrieval system, or transmitted, in any form or by any means, without prior written permission of the publisher, or, in Canada, in the case of photocopying or other reprographic copying, a licence from Access Copyright, www.accesscopyright.ca.

20 19 18 17 16 15 14 13 12 11   5 4 3 2 1

Printed in Canada on FSC-certified ancient-forest-free paper
(100% post-consumer recycled) that is processed chlorine- and acid-free.

Library and Archives Canada Cataloguing in Publication

Feminist ethics and social policy: towards a new global political economy of care / edited by Rianne Mahon and Fiona Robinson.

Includes bibliographical references and index.
Also issued in electronic format.
ISBN 978-0-7748-2105-6 (bound); ISBN 978-0-7748-2106-3 (pbk.)

1. Women household employees. 2. Women caregivers. 3. Women foreign workers. 4. Social policy – Moral and ethical aspects. 5. Transnationalism – Social aspects. 6. Feminist ethics. I. Mahon, Rianne. II. Robinson, Fiona

HQ1155.F44 2011   331.4'8164   C2011-903544-8

e-book ISBNs: 978-0-7748-2107-0 (pdf); 978-0-7748-2108-7 (epub)

Canadä

UBC Press gratefully acknowledges the financial support for our publishing program of the Government of Canada (through the Canada Book Fund), the Canada Council for the Arts, and the British Columbia Arts Council.

This book has been published with the help of a grant from the Canadian Federation for the Humanities and Social Sciences, through the Aid to Scholarly Publications Program, using funds provided by the Social Sciences and Humanities Research Council of Canada.

Printed and bound in Canada by Friesens
Set in Futura Condensed and Warnock by Artegraphica Design Co. Ltd.
Copy editor: Joanne Richardson
Proofreader: Dianne Tiefensee
Indexer: Lillian Ashworth

UBC Press
The University of British Columbia
2029 West Mall
Vancouver, BC V6T 1Z2
www.ubcpress.ca

Contents

Abbreviations / vii

Introduction / 1
RIANNE MAHON AND FIONA ROBINSON

Part 1: The Transnational Movement of Care

1 Towards a Transnational Analysis of the Political Economy of Care / 21
FIONA WILLIAMS

2 Migration and Globalized Care Work: The Case of Internationally Educated Nurses in Canada / 39
CHRISTINA GABRIEL

3 The Global Migration of Care Labour: Filipino Workers in Japan / 60
HIRONORI ONUKI

Part 2: Transnational Influence of Care Discourses

4 Transnationalizing (Child) Care Policy: The OECD and the World Bank / 77
RIANNE MAHON

5 Social Investment Policy in South Korea / 94
ITO PENG

6 Reimagined Intimate Relations: Elder and Child Care in Japan since the 1990s / 111
YUKI TSUJI

Part 3: The Transnational Ethics of Care

7 Care Ethics and the Transnationalization of Care: Reflections on Autonomy, Hegemonic Masculinities, and Globalization / 127
FIONA ROBINSON

8 The Dark Side of Care: The Push Factors of Human Trafficking / 145
OLENA HANKIVSKY

9 A Feminist Democratic Ethics of Care and Global Care Workers: Citizenship and Responsibility / 162
JOAN C. TRONTO

Conclusion: Integrating the Ethics and Social Politics of Care / 178
RIANNE MAHON AND FIONA ROBINSON

Notes / 184

References / 191

Contributors / 217

Index / 220

Abbreviations

AOTS	Association for Overseas Technical Scholarship
CAN	Canadian Nurses Association
CEC	Canadian Experience Class
CERI	Centre for Educational Research and Innovation (OECD)
CIC	Citizenship and Immigration Canada
CIHI	Canadian Institute for Health Information
CIS	Commonwealth of Independent States
DELSA	Directorate for Employment, Labour and Social Affairs (OECD)
ECC	early childhood care
ECD	early child development
ECE	early childhood education
ECEC	early child education and care
EPA	Economic Partnership Agreement
EWL	European Women's Lobby
GOL	General Occupations List
HRSDC	Human Resources and Skills Development Canada
IENs	Internationally Educated Nurses

ILO	International Labour Organization
IMF	International Monetary Fund
INGOs	international non-governmental organizations
IOs	international organizations
IRPA	Immigration Reform and Protection Act
JICWEL	Japan International Corporation of Welfare Services
JPEPA	Japan-Philippines Economic Partnership Agreement
KWDI	Korean Women's Development Institute
LCP	Live-In Caregiver Program
LFCAJ	Licensed Filipino Caregivers Association in Japan
LTCI	long-term care insurance
MOEHRD	Ministry of Education and Human Resource Development (Korea)
MHLW	Ministry of Health, Labour and Welfare (Japan)
NIKKEIREN	Japan Federation of Employers' Association
ODA	Official Development Assistance
OECD	Organization for Economic Cooperation and Development
OJT	on-the-job training
PNPs	provincial nominee programs
RENGO	Japanese Trade Union Confederation
RNs	registered nurses
RNAO	Registered Nurses' Association of Ontario
ROWITE	role of women in the economy
SAPs	structural adjustment programs
TFWP	Temporary Foreign Worker Program
TPV	Tropical Paradise Village (Philippines)
UNDP	United Nations Development Program
UNESCO	United Nations Educational, Scientific and Cultural Organization
UNFPA	United Nations Population Fund
UNICEF	United Nations Children's Fund

FEMINIST ETHICS AND SOCIAL POLICY

Introduction

RIANNE MAHON AND FIONA ROBINSON

The term "care" has two related meanings. The first refers to a set of activities and form of labour focused on social reproduction, including child care, elder care, care for the sick and those with disabilities as well as other forms of household and domestic labour. The second involves the understanding of care as the basis for a system of ethics. In Virginia Held's (2006, 10) words, the central focus of the ethics of care is on "the compelling moral salience of attending to and meeting the needs of particular others for whom we take responsibility." One of the main aims of this book is to elucidate the theoretical and practical relationship between aspects of care that have, for the most part, been treated separately, that is, the ethics of care, developments in the social politics of care, and the impact of transnationalization, including the formation of a "global care chain" (Hochschild 2000).

Bringing together the ethics and social politics of care is, however, a challenging task. It has been suggested that, in focusing on care *ethics*, care as "nurturance" is inevitably foregrounded, thus excluding other non-relational aspects of social reproduction, such as cleaning and food preparation. By privileging relational, face-to-face caring practices, we simultaneously privilege the experience of white women and exclude large numbers of very-low-wage workers, thus excluding the experiences of women of colour and poor women (Duffy 2005, 79). In this book, we use a broad definition of care – one that includes nurturant care and other social reproductive activities. In so doing, we take seriously Duffy's challenge to "think broadly about ways to bring together current work on nurturance with ... literature on reproductive labor ... to create a more inclusive and nuanced model of the very complex interactions between care and inequalities" (80-81). To this end, our approach eschews idealized or essentialized normative arguments about women's care in favour of a critical political ethics of care that interrogates the patriarchal and often neocolonial conditions under which values and practices associated with caring have developed in and across societies.

An ethics of care that is political and critical must be grounded in the concrete activities of real people in the context of webs of social relations. In turn, these webs are affected by politics and the structure of social policies. In most OECD countries, social policy structures are neither "frozen" nor melting under the influence of neoliberal restructuring; rather, social policy discourses highlight the growing need for non-familial care arrangements associated with women's rising labour force participation rates and the demographics of aging societies. Needs do not, however, speak for themselves (Fraser 1989a); rather, it is the politics of needs – and the power relations they reflect – that determines which needs are placed on the public agenda.

In the past, the politics of needs was played out largely within national contexts and reflected the existing balance of power therein. This is less true today, however. First, international organizations like the Organization for Economic Cooperation and Development (OECD) and the World Bank have come to play an increasingly important role in coordinating policy responses. Second, as feminist scholars have documented, care needs in the richer countries are being increasingly met by the prodigious flow of female labour from poorer countries. This volume aims to interrogate the implications of these transnational flows of people and ideas. Thus, while it includes careful analysis of actual policy developments in particular national contexts, it also includes innovative theorizations of gender and race relations, global justice and neocolonialism, and care and masculinities as they relate to the development of a global ethics and social politics of care.

We choose the term "transnationalization" rather than the more popular "globalization" to avoid the latter's association with universalism. To the extent that "global" refers to the stretching of phenomena – including social relations – across the world as a whole, it does not capture important disparities and regional concentrations in the nature and direction of flows of people, responsibilities, and resources associated with care. Moreover, as is evident in many of the chapters in this book, the state remains a crucial actor in the regulation and promotion of transnationalized care.

In this chapter, we review important developments in the ethics of care and then discuss the "discovery of care" in the field of comparative social policy. This forms the basis for an integrated discussion of the ethics and politics of care in a globalizing world.

The Ethics of Care

While care work in the global economy was becoming increasingly commodified and transnationalized, a then unrelated development was occurring within the academic fields of moral psychology, ethics, and feminist theory. In the 1970s, Nancy Chodorow's (1974, 8) pathbreaking work challenged the masculine bias of psychoanalytic theory by arguing that the existence of sex differences in early development does not mean that women have "weaker" ego boundaries than men but, rather, that girls come to experience themselves as more continuous with, and related to, the external object-world and to others. Moreover, Chodorow argued that difference cannot be put down to anatomy or any other essential quality but, rather, to the reality that, universally, women are largely responsible for early child care. In 1980, as Virginia Held (2006, 26) points out, before Sarah Ruddick's important essay "Maternal Thinking" (1980) was published, there was virtually no philosophical acknowledgment that mothers think or reason, or that one can find moral values in this practice. Two year's later, Carol Gilligan's seminal book, *In a Different Voice*, used empirical research from developmental psychology – much influenced by Chodorow's work on object-relations theory – to address gender differences in moral development.

It was Gilligan who first gave us the language of the "ethics of care" – an approach to morality that fundamentally challenges the dominance of universalist or rule-based approaches to ethics. Where dominant views of ethics centre on the rights and obligations of autonomous moral agents, the ethics of care presents a vision of morality that requires an understanding of context and an ontology of relationality or mutualism. From this perspective, moral dilemmas are less about "contests of rights" and more about ways of ensuring that "everyone will be responded to and included; that no one will be left alone or hurt" (Gilligan 1982, 59-63). Thus, morality and the preservation of life are contingent on recognizing and sustaining connection and taking responsibility for others by keeping the web of relationships intact, while remaining cognizant of the issue of rights (59).

Since the first publication of *In a Different Voice*, there has been a remarkable proliferation of research on the ethics of care in moral and political philosophy and feminist theory. Ruddick, Held, and Noddings are widely regarded as the most important "first-generation" care theorists (Ruddick 1980, 1989; Held 1993; Noddings 1984). Despite their influence on the direction of ethics and feminist theory, all three have been criticized for their moral foundationalism, their personalized or parochial view of caring, and for essentializing the role of women as carers. While debating these particular charges is beyond the scope of this introduction, it is worth noting that these critiques raise important areas for concern regarding the dangers of idealizing, feminizing, and personalizing care ethics. The contributors to this volume are acutely aware of these potential problems. They argue convincingly that caring relations must be understood as shaped and constrained by relations of power, including those in the global political economy. Moreover, a *feminist* ethics of care problematizes and challenges naturalized or essentialist assumptions regarding women and caregiving. It also addresses the wider structural and normative reasons – as found in the global political economy and in social constructions of masculinity and femininity – for the concentration of women in care work (see Robinson, Tronto, and Williams, this volume).

In spite of these alleged shortcomings, the important work of early ethicists paved the way for the development of care ethics, both in their own work and in the work of those who followed (see Held 2006). "Second-generation" care theorists, including Joan Tronto and Selma Sevenhuijsen, sought to overcome the dangers of essentialism, parochialism, and paternalism by "politicizing" care ethics. Thus, by the mid-1990s, the debate had moved towards exploring the relationship between care and the practices of democracy and citizenship. Importantly, this work took a critical stance by addressing inequalities in the giving and receiving of care based on gender, race, and class (Tronto 1993; Sevenhuijsen 1998). Moreover, critical feminist theorists in international relations sought to address the relevance of care ethics for global politics, employing care ethics as a critical lens rather than as a normative ideal (Hutchings 2000; Robinson 1999, 2006b).

A special issue of *Hypatia* on "Feminist Ethics and Social Policy" (1995) was dedicated to considering the ways in which the ethics of care could serve as both an ethical framework for, and moral lens through which to view, issues of social policy. As Patrice DiQuinzio and Iris Young, editors of the issue, argue: "if feminist ethics has indeed mobilized important paradigm shifts in normative analysis, then this should enable creative ways of reflection on social policy" (DiQuinzio and Young 1995, 1). Articles in this issue address a diverse range of institutional arenas of social policy, including specific policy and legislative acts concerning fathers' rights, family and medical leave, immigration, and race classification. While there is diversity in the approaches to feminist ethics developed among the contributors, there is widespread agreement on the need for contextualization in both ethical theory and social policy in terms of the specificity and complexity of the sociocultural contexts in which policy issues arise (4).

A number of other authors – including many of the contributors to this volume – have taken up the challenge of integrating care ethics and social policy. For example, while primarily interested in social policy, Fiona Williams is fully committed to elucidating the values – arising from an ethics of care – that underwrite her policy prescriptions. Indeed, she convincingly argues that, if care policies are going to fulfill their innovative potential in ways that secure greater and not less equality, then the political values that support such policies have to be clear (Williams 2001, 473). To that end, she develops a "new political ethics of care" that invites a robust discussion of the values that are important to people in their relationships of care and intimacy. In particular, Williams is cognizant of the "shifting relations and changing boundaries in care practices and provision," which demand that we address issues surrounding disability, "race," and migration – all of which raise particular challenges in conceptualizing care in the contemporary context (468).

Similarly, while Joan Tronto's starting point for considering care is political theory and philosophy, her work has always been grounded in a consideration of the "real world" of care provision. Indeed, as she and Julie White argue, both "rights" and "needs" discourses are limited by their formalistic approach to the relationship between care and justice, needs and rights. In contrast, they suggest that an exploration of these relationships must begin with the "actually existing organization of care and justice" – in particular, the invisibility of care to some, and the inaccessibility of rights to others (White and Tronto 2004, 426). Finally, Olena Hankivsky's *Social Policy and the Ethic of Care* focuses on the question "what are the consequences for the human need for care in social policy" (Hankivsky 2004, 1-2). She, too, notices the gap between theoretical and public policy analysis and seeks to address it through her study of issues and institutions in Canadian public policy.

In many ways, the politicization of care ethics by contemporary care theorists has meant that a consideration of the policy implications of care ethics unavoidably becomes important. For example, Selma Sevenhuijsen's

Citizenship and the Ethics of Care demonstrates how, by locating the ethics of care within notions of citizenship, care is brought into public debates without being associated with a fixed caring identity or foundational claims about "moral goodness" (Sevenhuijsen 1998, 15). This theoretical argument then leads to an analysis of care and justice in debates on child custody, and to a case study of feminist ethics and public health-care policies in the Netherlands.

This book is the result of our commitment to furthering this dialogue between feminist ethicists and analysts of social policy. While most of its contributors would situate themselves primarily in one or another of these fields of research, all are aware of the need for conversation across what is sometimes regarded as a "divide" between "theory" and "policy." Only when policy analysis is fully cognizant of the ethical implications of its recommendations can it lead to policy making and implementation that furthers feminist goals by taking care and social reproduction seriously.

Social Policy: The Discovery of Care

Social policy research traditionally focused on transfers – social insurance (e.g., pensions, unemployment insurance), child and family benefits, social assistance. While earlier research was concerned to explain the rise of the welfare state as a consequence of industrialization and urbanization, attention turned to accounting for differences in the pattern of welfare state expenditure. Building on the class-centred politics of power resource theory, in the 1990s Esping-Andersen's (1990) *Three Worlds of Welfare Capitalism* – liberal, social democratic, and conservative-corporatist – became the focal point of much of the debate. It was feminist researchers, however, who uncovered the silent gendered assumptions governing social reproduction via the unpaid work of women in the home. Thus McIntosh (1978, 264) argues as follows:

> For the reproduction of labour power the state sustains a family household system in which a number of people are dependent for financial support on the wages of a few adult members, primarily of a male breadwinner, and in which they are all dependent for cleaning, food preparation and so forth on the unpaid work done chiefly by a woman. At the same time, the state itself carries out some of these functions of financial support and of servicing; yet it usually does so under such ideological conditions that it is seen as "taking over" functions properly belonging to the family or as "substituting" for work that "should be done by a housewife."

While McIntosh was criticized for generalizing from the UK experience (Jenson 1986), subsequent feminist scholarship began to develop typologies of gendered welfare regimes. Thus Lewis and Ostner (1991) distinguish between strong, moderate, and weak male breadwinner models, while Sainsbury (1996) contrasts the male breadwinner model to one in which access to benefits was based according to individual entitlement.

Yet, even as the social policy implications of women's unpaid domestic caregiving role were being uncovered, women were entering (and remaining in) the paid labour force in rising numbers. This happened earlier and more extensively in countries like Sweden, Denmark, Canada, and the United States, where women's labour force participation rates are now nearly as high as men's, but pressures for change are being felt in all OECD countries. This has given rise to what Lister (1994) and McLaughlin and Glendinning (1994) call the "defamilialization" of care, a concept later adopted by Esping-Andersen (1999). That is, if women are no longer available to provide care for the very young, the frail elderly, or those with disabilities on an unpaid basis in the home, those care needs will have to be met from other sources – state, market, and/or community sector. Defamilialization has, in turn, been associated with the monetization of care (Antonnen, Sipilä, and Baldock 2003, 177).

Monetization has not, however, necessarily entailed the commodification of care. Monetization involves payment of wages and salaries to care workers, but access to care services is structured by the rules of citizenship. In other words, there is a right to publicly financed (and often publicly provided) care. Commodification accompanies monetization when access to (paid) care is made through the market. In many ways, moreover, caring labour resists commodification. For example, not only does caring labour clearly entail a large "noncommodified human element" (Radin 1996, 105), but this element is made more complex by the human relationships that are involved. Furthermore, as Himmelweit (2008, 350) argues:

> without lowering standards, the productivity of caring cannot be raised substantially through mass production ... because caring, as well as performing physical activity, is the development of a relationship between a carer and the person cared for. This limits how many people can be cared for at the same time ... Indeed, what in other industries would be seen as measures of high productivity are specifically taken as indices of low quality when it comes to care.

For instance, high child-staff ratios are generally considered an indicator of lower quality of child care. Without public support, however, the service is too expensive for most families to afford, giving rise to a trade-off between affordability and wages that are in line with those in other sectors in the national economy. According to Esping-Andersen (1999), different countries have addressed the dilemma in different ways.[1] In social democratic welfare regimes, the state finances and often provides social-care services; in liberal regimes, tax incentives can be used to cheapen the cost of commercial care for some while others rely on low-wage informal (non-regulated) care; and in conservative continental regimes, the growth of monetized care is stunted. Antonnen and Sipilä (1996), however, distinguish between the familial care model found in Portugal, Spain, Greece, and Italy and the central European subsidiarity model, where, while formal responsibility remains with the family, the state subsidizes production by religious and political organizations.

In a later five-country study, however, Antonnen, Sipilä, and Baldock (2003, 171) are more cautious about the existence of nationwide care regimes. They find that the five countries studied – Finland, Germany, the United States, the United Kingdom, and Japan – all exhibit considerable geographic and sectoral diversity. They also rightly stress the importance of change. On the one hand, demographic pressures – aging populations, falling fertility rates – are putting pressure on "laggard" countries like Germany (Henninger, Wimbauer, and Dombrowski 2008), Japan (Tsuji, this volume), and Korea (Peng, this volume) to support the defamilialization of care. On the other hand, fiscal constraints have prompted the move by the United Kingdom to introduce vouchers for elder care (Ungerson and Yeandle 2007), while another European study finds the proliferation of schemes to support the purchase of home-based child (and elder) care (Lister et al. 2007). Although Sweden has proven more resistant to the growth of home-based child care, it has accepted the creation of a (publicly subsidized) market especially for elder care, in which those seeking care can choose between for-profit, non-profit, and public providers.

Demographic and other pressures, of course, do not dictate change. Politics, including the politics of ideas or discourse, shape the way new needs are understood and the directions in which solutions are sought. Thus, supranational (the European Union) and international organizations have been actively encouraging the adoption of measures to promote the "reconciliation of work and family life." The doctrine of new public management, which the OECD helped to spread, provided the rationale for

Sweden's opening to private (including for-profit) care provision, but the creation of a market for child care was actively promoted by neoliberal elements within Sweden and by the union representing the majority of elder and child-care givers, which felt that its members could secure higher wages if there were more competition among providers. In the United Kingdom, disability rights activists have strongly supported the move to choice (Williams 2001). The construction of a broader discourse of care can also be used to construct alliances between those needing various forms of care and those involved in its provision (Folbre 2008).

This takes us back to the question of the link between social policy and the ethics of care. While social policy research has focused on cross-national comparisons, feminist researchers have not ignored ethical questions such as those raised around the issue of "autonomy." Thus Orloff (1993) and O'Connor (1993) stress the importance of policies that promote women's capacity to form autonomous households, while a similar concern underpins feminist interest in the concept of defamilialization.[2] Lewis puts the issue starkly: "If care is a universal human need ... it has to be possible for anyone to choose to do it, as a matter of both principle and pragmatic policy making. For, given that informal care usually involves emotion and love as well as labour and passive 'watching over' ... policy must make it possible to exercise what Sen ... terms 'real agency freedom' – a genuine choice to do care work" (Lewis 2008, 276).

While autonomy is recognized as an important feminist goal, feminist ethicists are aware of the dangers of emphasizing traditional masculinist conceptions of autonomy at the expense of relationality. When "autonomy" refers to isolated, self-reliant moral selves it does not adequately reflect social reality in most communities around the world. Feminists have argued that one of the effects of this ontology has been to obscure from view the particular experiences of women, who are most likely to define themselves in and through their relations with children and other family members – including the elderly or chronically ill – or with friends or members of their communities. Indeed, the picture of "autonomous man" distorts not just the experiences of women: all people live lives that are, at least during some periods of time, interdependent with those of others.

From the perspective of "relational autonomy," it becomes clear that there is more than one agent seeking "autonomy" and that, ultimately, autonomy is achieved in and through relationships. As Antonnen and Sipilä (1996, 90) put it, "putting the issue of personal autonomy at the centre of social services highlights the perspective of women, but autonomy is also important to the people who use services, such as frail elderly people and disabled people." Thus, as both Williams (2001) and Daly (2002) suggest, we need to think about how social policy arrangements can respect and serve both care receivers and care providers.

Transnationalization of Care

For the most part, social policy analysts, including feminists, have focused on cross-national comparisons, ignoring not only important differences within regimes (Antonnen, Sipilä, and Baldock 2003) but also the increasingly permeable (to flows of people and ideas as well as to capital) character of such national boundaries. Likewise, after breaking free from the received view that care pertains only to personal relations within the "private sphere," the ethics of care has, until recently, also assumed a national setting. As Nancy Fraser notes of her classic 1997 essay on models of care, "like all my welfare work in those years, the article implicitly assumed that the ideal post-industrial feminist welfare state would be located in a bounded political community that corresponded to a territorial state" (Fraser 2008, 229). Yet, as Yeates (2005, 232) notes, "the treatment of 'national' care regimes as enclosed entities decontextualized from the global political economy in which they are embedded, is no longer justifiable, if it ever was. Unequal relations within the household similarly have to be situated within an international division of reproductive labour that is structured by social class, 'race'/ethnicity, and 'gender inequalities'" (ibid.). The social politics and ethics of care, in other words, have to be situated within a setting that is increasingly global – from "care chains" that can span the globe to travelling social policy discourses.

One aspect of the transnationalization of care is the flow of social policy discourse, in which international organizations like the OECD and the World Bank are playing a critical role. Initially, both organizations helped to disseminate the view that the welfare state was a burden and had to be cut back in the name of growth and international competitiveness. As Mahon (this volume) documents, this discourse has changed (somewhat) in recognition that there is a role for the "right" social policies – that is, those that reflect the "social investment" paradigm (Jenson, 2007). Peck and Theodore (2008) show that these organizations have not only looked to the global North for new "best practices": the much touted "conditional cash transfers" were developed in and by Latin American experts, especially from Mexico.

Advice offered OECD member countries on measures to reconcile work and family life has come to incorporate more of a gender equality perspective and, as such, if implemented, would go a long way towards addressing the care deficit in the North. The new social policy discourses of the World Bank also reflect the impact of international feminism. Yet, as Bedford's (2009, 198) study of the World Bank shows, this has involved "measures to strengthen the family as an informal institution necessary to reduce poverty." Moreover, Molyneux (2006) documents the ways that the new conditional cash transfers have involved the imposition of new caring obligations on women in the South, while Rosemberg (2006, 75) argues that, in Brazil, the Bank's child-care projects "have encouraged programs ... with low state investment, low quality services and the inadequate remuneration of women's labor. Thus they reinforce the ideology of traditional family values, which create and sustain the dominance of gender, class, race and age."

The second dimension of the transnationalization of care has to do with the intensification of global care chains. The growing "care crisis" (Daly and Lewis 2000) arising from inadequate political responses to the defamilialization of care provides part of the explanation for the growth of global care chains. The flow of (mainly women) caregivers from poorer countries to wealthier countries offers a low-wage solution to the dilemma posed by the trade-off between affordability and fair wages for caregivers and the failure to get men to share care responsibilities. This is not happening spontaneously; rather, it is being aided by the state-sponsored spread of such solutions in Western Europe, often fuelled by a mix of still-hegemonic mother-substitute "ideals of care" and immigration regimes that facilitate such flows (Lister et al. 2007, 161). American researchers have shown the heavy reliance of US families on (documented and undocumented) women migrants from South America and elsewhere (Hondagneu-Sotelo 2001; Parreñas 2001a; Ehrenreich and Hochschild 2003), while, in Canada, the domestic Live-In Caregiver Program has attracted critical attention (Bakan and Stasiulis 1997; Spitzer et al. 2003). Migrant carers are also being drawn to the Middle East and the Far East, including societies, like Japan, that have hitherto remained relatively closed to immigrants (Onuki this volume).

As Arat-Koc (2006, 87) argues, such refamilialization of care has the effect of hiding once again the costs of social reproduction: "For employers of domestic workers, it is often the neo-liberal ethics and expectations of the contemporary workplace for many professionals, while for the domestic worker/caregiver, it is the requirements of live-in arrangements and immigration restrictions associated with temporary or undocumented status, which force both groups of women to tuck their maternal roles neatly away, out of sight and out of mind, from the market and the society they are living in." This solution is eerily reminiscent of Nancy Folbre's "CorporNation," in which citizenship is extended only to adults under fifty who are well-educated, physically and emotionally healthy, have no children, and are without responsibilities for the care of others (e.g., elderly parents). Citizenship is withdrawn from those who no longer meet these stringent criteria (Folbre 2006). Yet, as Hochschild (2000, 136) notes, the (invisible) global care chain on which such an adult earner family has come to rely often connects "three sets of care-takers – one cares for the migrant's children back home, a second cares for the children of the woman who cares for the migrant's children, and a third, the migrating mother herself, cares for the [children of] professionals in the First World."

Parreñas (2001a) spells out some of the consequences for migrant caregivers. They are entangled in what amounts to transnational families, in which intimacy is expected (and often given) to care receivers in rich countries, while they are forced to offer "love by remittance" to their own. Many are also caught in contradictory class locations: trained as teachers and nurses at home, they experience downward mobility as domestic caregivers in the receiving country. For instance, the wages of a domestic worker in Hong Kong are fifteen times the amount Filipinas can earn as school teachers at home (Ehrenreich and Hochschild 2003, 8). Finally, migrant caregivers are reduced to partial citizenship as immigration laws (and racism) mean they are neither fully integrated in receiving nations nor adequately protected by their own governments (Parreñas 2001a, 37).

Clearly, poverty in their home countries and the broader global inequalities that produce it play a crucial part in pushing migrant care workers. So, too, do the policies of their governments, a reflection of what Sassen (2002a, 265) calls the "feminization of survival": "Not only are households, indeed whole communities, increasingly dependent on women for their survival, but so too are governments, along with enterprises that function on the margins of the legal economy." Thus, the Philippine government has played an active part in promoting the migration of Filipinas as an important source of remittances and, as Onuki (this volume) shows, skill acquisition.

While the concept of a global care chain has helped to highlight the increasingly transnational character of care provision, the original concept has been criticized for focusing too narrowly on the refamilialization of care. In particular, Yeates (2004, 379) argues for broadening the concept to recognize (1) different levels in skill and occupational hierarchies occupied by the migrants; (2) different family situations; (3) work in institutional as well as household settings; and (4) different types of care, including health, education, and sexual services. We concur. Thus, the chapters by Gabriel and Onuki look at the complex arrangements surrounding the migration of nurses to Canada (Gabriel) and Japan (Onuki). As the latter's analysis suggests, it is also important to recognize that, while women constitute the majority of migrant care workers, men too are involved.

Some of the literature on the global care chain also downplays the caregivers' own agency. Yet, educated women (and men) in countries like Mexico and the Philippines may seek posts abroad not simply to improve their families' situation but also to escape from a "stalled gender revolution" (Parreñas 2003) at home. Migration may offer a way out of obligations to provide care for elderly in-laws or of having to defer to abusive men (Erhenreich and Hochschild 2003, 11). Resistance to the limitations of their partial citizenship can take informal expression – for example, the use of days off to assert cultural rights in public spaces – as well as more overt demands on their home governments to protect their rights or on the host government to recognize their "right to hospitality" (Sarvasy and Longo 2004, 404).

This raises the broader question: who are the subjects of rights in the contemporary world? As Fraser (2008, 232) now recognizes, "the new salience of transnational politics and claims-making, ranging from human rights activism to international feminist and to the World Social Forum has problematized the national answer to the question of 'who.'" More broadly, Sarvasy and Longo (2004, 396) call for a multi-scalar citizenship: "First, world citizenship must be nestled in and supported by host nation citizenship. Second, world citizenship must be sustained by what we call 'deterritorialized citizenship,' the actualization of citizenship rights outside the territory of the state. Third, the practices of care in the household must be seen as entailing the negotiations of different levels of citizenship." These critiques point to the fact that traditional concepts of rights, justice, and citizenship may be inadequate to address the contemporary challenges of care and well-being at the transnational scale.

To be sure, the increasing intensity and scale of transnational care chains has given rise to a wider debate about their rights. Thus, in 1990 the UN General Assembly passed the International Convention on the Protection of the Rights of All Migrant Workers and Members of Their Families – but Canada, the United States, and many Western European countries refused to sign it (Arat-Koc 2006, 79). More recently (2003), the UN established the

Global Commission on International Migration at the request of the secretary general and Sweden, Switzerland, Brazil, Morocco, and the Philippines.

While it might seem obvious that an ethics of care is best suited to illuminate these issues, this is not reflected in the discourse of states and multilateral organizations. As Mahon (this volume) points out, the dominant normative discourses, especially those directed at countries of the global South by international organizations, tend to foreground the "rights of the child" as well as traditional understandings of "gender equality," which rely heavily on rights language. Yet, as many of the chapters in this volume demonstrate, the ethical language of care can speak to the relationality – itself often characterized by an uneven distribution of power – of care work in ways that moral rights language cannot (see Robinson, this volume). While gender equality promotion – especially programs focused on "women's empowerment" in the global South – has concentrated on getting women into paid employment, it has often overlooked the issue of unremunerated reproductive labour and the "double burden" that exists for many women. Furthermore, when this dilemma has been recognized, solutions are often aimed at encouraging men to be more active and better carers within the family. Not only does this promote a limited vision of the family and sexuality – what Bedford calls "caring couplehood" – but it also ends up endorsing a completely privatized solution to the "social reproduction dilemma and erasing childcare provision as a priority" (Bedford 2008, 93).

Conclusion

One of the aims of this book is to build upon the important work of scholars like Sevenhuijsen in light of crucial changes in the nature and structure of care work within the last decade, while integrating these insights with those drawn from the social policy literature. Specifically, we begin from the premise that the commodification and transnationalization of care creates new and unprecedented challenges for considering the ethics and social politics of care. Transnational, commodified care is now a defining feature of the global political economy. These developments raise ethical and policy challenges related to migration, citizenship, and labour as well as basic political and moral concepts like equality, exclusion, and democracy. Indeed, it may be that the paradigm of distributive justice – so dominant in normative political philosophy since the 1970s – is inadequate to address the complexities of globalized care. As Sevenhuijsen (1998, 86) argues: "Care is, after all, not simply a matter of distributing 'goods and services'; it has to do primarily with quality of life, and how we experience and interpret this. It also has to do with the ways in which power processes are involved in this context." Moreover, on the policy side, analysis of care-related policies demonstrates that economic lenses, through which public policy is so often framed, are wholly inadequate when "juxtaposed with the moral and social aspects of care policy" (Daly 2002, 269). Care is not just about money or services: it is also about time. Care policy must address the needs and agents not just of individuals but also of both the givers and the receivers of care. Finally, public policy on care also connects in fundamental ways with values and norms and the organization of society itself, including dimensions of gender equality and the legitimization of care in societies (268).

While care work involves more than child care, many of the chapters in this volume focus on national regimes and transnational policy discourses relating to child care. This is not surprising, given the enormous and very visible rise in migrant child-care labour around the world. In thinking ethically about this new "international reproductive division of labour" (Parreñas 2000), care theorists must be especially cognizant of the need to challenge, rather than to valorize, visions of child care that reinforce stereotypes of gender, race, and class as well as relations of care that are potentially or actually exploitative, abusing, demeaning, or otherwise unfair (Carse and Lindemann Nelson 1996, 20).

Furthermore, these developments push moral theorists and social policy analysts to challenge the notion that domestic work can be understood as a relationship between "private women." Guest domestic worker programs connect affluent states with inadequate social provision for care and poorer states with labour export policies (Sarvasy and Longo 2004, 409). Precisely because it is now negotiated by states, the global interdependence of care demands a multi-scalar feminist politics of care. This volume recognizes the importance of understanding both the "fundamental importance of state policies and ideologies that govern and interpret the social position and meaning of both care work and care workers" and the way these state policies are mutually constitutive of transnational institutions and discourses (Litt and Zimmerman 2003, 157).

While the trend towards migrant women working as "nannies" in income-rich countries is highly visible, "maids and sex workers," as well as nurses, elder-care workers, and teachers, should be considered alongside child-care workers as part of the "feminization of survival" (Sassen 2002). These "counter-geographies of globalization" – which include labour migration for domestic work and highly regulated industries such as nursing as well as the illegal trafficking in women for the sex industry – are of growing importance as profit-making activities, including as sources of revenue for some governments in often deeply indebted countries.

While early care ethicists often valorized the activities of caring, these developments uncover the "dark side" of care (Hankivsky, this volume). Thinking ethically about women in the sex industry alongside analyses of nannies and domestic labour raises important moral questions about the commodification of women's bodies and the role of norms of masculinity in sustaining and reproducing these patterns of "women's work" in the global economy (Robinson, this volume).

Rather than idealizing caring relations, a contemporary political ethics of care must address the moral and political implications of the global care crises as they are manifested both globally and locally. Ad hoc, exploitative, and excessively privatized solutions to the question of how we will care for each other are woefully inadequate in the current social, economic, and demographic contexts. Care ethics can serve as a lens through which to focus and organize our thinking about the ways in which care is delivered at the local, national, and global levels. To do so effectively, however, it must confront head on the realities of human vulnerability and dependence, and of our embodied, fragile, interdependent selves. With the recognition of this vulnerability comes a renewed awareness of the empowering potential of human relations and mutuality, of the tenacity of our struggles to enhance and foster our interdependence, and of the need to continue to care for one another in the face of the most severe forms of hardship. As geographer Victoria Lawson (2007, 1) argues, care ethics focuses our attention on the social and how it is constructed through equal power relationships, but it also moves us beyond critique and towards the construction of new forms of relationships, institutions, and action that enhance mutuality and well-being.

Finally, one of the principal objectives of this volume is to bring to bear insights drawn from both the ethics and the social politics of care on the transnationalization of care. As we have seen, there are bridges upon which we can build. Feminist theorists like Joan Tronto and Margaret Walker point to the importance of the power relations underlying care arrangements – relations that operate at the macro as well as at the micro scale. At the same time, social policy analysts like Williams, Daly, and Lewis highlight the normative implications of different social policy designs. One key area in which the two approaches come together is around the importance of ideas or discourses of care. Thus, a number of our contributors from both traditions stress the importance of ways of framing the case for care – the right to be cared for as an autonomous person and the right to give (or not to give) care on terms that value the activity of caring – as a fundamental component of citizenship at multiple scales.

PART 1

The Transnational Movement of Care

Towards a Transnational Analysis of the Political Economy of Care

FIONA WILLIAMS

The resurgence of the employment of domestic and care workers in private homes in many industrialized countries over the last two decades has been shaped by important social changes, most notable among which are the increased responsibilities and rights of women across the globe to be both earners and carers. This reflects the graduated shifts from the "male-breadwinner" to the "adult-worker" model that are taking place in many industrialized societies as well as the unemployment and poverty in developing countries. As many of those who carry out this work are migrant women, this reveals the movement of women seeking opportunities created by the changing patterns of postcolonial migration to financially support their families. Such migrations are also structured by the policies developed by richer nation-states. The nature of care regimes in host countries clearly influences take up: where care provision is commodified and where care cultures favour home-based/surrogate care, reliance on the low-paid end of the private market is more common (Ungerson and Yeandle 2007; Williams and Gavanas 2008). At the same time, migration rules construct the legal, social, and civil rights of migrants in different ways, in tandem with employment policies that may serve to deregulate the economy and to increase the casualization of labour. Superimposed on this universe of change is the ongoing reconstitution of social relations of gender, care, and domestic service; of hierarchies of ethnicity and nationality; and of differentiated meanings of, and rights to, citizenship. This chapter draws on earlier research into migration and home-based care in Europe as a basis for developing a transnational analysis of the political economy of care (Lister et al. 2007, 137-65; Williams and Gavanas 2008; Williams 2007; Williams, Tobio, and Gavanas 2009; Williams, in press).

Different Levels of Analysis

In the description given above, it is possible to identify three interrelated levels of analysis. At the micro level are the everyday experiences of the relationship between migrant workers and their employers and/or those for whom they care; at the meso level is the national/supranational institutional context of those policies and practices that shape this everyday relationship; and at the macro level are the processes of globalization that have fostered a global political economy of care. The concept of the "global care chain" (Parreñas 2001a; Ehrenreich and Hochschild 2003) exemplifies the link between the micro and macro levels. It refers to the migration of women from poorer regions of the world to work as carers for the children, households, or older family members of employed women in the West in order to support their own children, whom they leave in the care of female relatives in their countries of origin. At the macro level, female migration and what Parreñas calls an international division of reproductive labour (Parreñas 2001a, 61-79) provide opportunities for women from poorer countries to support their families.[1]

Research on the meso level has generally referred to national or transnational institutions, networks, or practices that sustain or constrain these processes of work, care, and migration. In the European context, however, the meso level has been extended to include state policies for care, employment, and migration (Williams and Gavanas 2008; Williams, in press). The global care chain emerged from research on the United States as the receiving country and, as such, identifies a lack of public care provision in shaping the demand for child and elder care. In Europe, however, it is not simply the absence of the state provision in care that shapes the demand for child and elder care and the supply of migrant care but, rather, the restructured nature of the state support that is available.

The last five years have seen the growing acceptance in many parts of Europe of child care as a public and not simply as a private responsibility (Lister et al. 2007). At the same time, the shift in a number of countries from providing care services (or, in the case of southern Europe, few services) to giving individuals cash payments to buy in-home-based care has shaped care provision for children as well as for older people and disabled people.

This might take the form of cash or tax credits or tax incentives to pay child minders, nannies, relatives, or domestic workers for their services. The United Kingdom, Spain, Finland, and France have all introduced some form of cash provision or tax credit to assist in buying help for child care in the home (Lister et al. 2007, 109-36), and Sweden has introduced tax breaks for people employing domestic help in the home. In the United Kingdom, for example, in an attempt to regularize private use of child carers, in 2006, tax credits were extended to the employment of registered nannies. There are also forms of "direct payments" that allow older people or disabled people to buy in-support and assistance (e.g., in the United Kingdom, Netherlands, Italy, and Austria) (Ungerson and Yeandle 2007; Bettio, Simonazzi, and Villa 2006). Both of these types of provision encourage the development of a particular form of home-based, often low-paid commodified care or domestic help, generally accessed privately through the market. This is where low-cost migrant labour steps in. Indeed, in Spain, Italy, and Greece, the strategy of employing migrant labour to meet care needs has become so prevalent that Bettio, Simonazzi, and Villa (2006, 272) describe it as a shift from a "family" model of care to a "migrant-in-the-family" model of care.

It is not only tax credits or allowances that shape demand and supply for home-based child care but also the way in which these legitimize the commodification of care. Research in Madrid and London (Williams and Gavanas 2008) found that the effect of these sorts of policies in countries where the private market dominates choices for child care was to position mothers as individual *consumers* choosing the right care for their children according to their care preferences. This is reinforced through the, now commonplace, use of unregulated paid domestic help in the home. In Madrid, where working mothers receive a small subsidy to help them purchase care, mothers felt it was their individual responsibility to find resources for child care in the private market. Day care in Britain is provided mainly through the market or voluntary sector; however, in spite of tax credits, nursery places are expensive, especially if parents have more than one child. Searching for value for money is what mothers find themselves doing in a marketized child-care economy. Williams (in press) argues that it is the ways these policies, practices, and social relations associated with care regimes dovetail in different ways with both those of migration regimes and employment regimes that contextualize the actions and experiences of migrant workers and their employers.

There are at least two reasons for identifying these mediating factors of nation-state (and, in some cases, EU) policy. The first is that they provide a basis for developing a cross-national analysis of why the employment of migrant care workers, while increasing in many European countries (Cancedda 2001), nevertheless varies between countries. Second, and more relevant for this chapter, this focus brings European welfare states into global perspective in that it reveals the ways in which, directly or indirectly, welfare societies may seek to reduce their social expenditure costs through migrant care labour. This allows us to extend the framework of analysis to bring in other forms of international reproductive labour, such as nurses, doctors, and teachers, a point that is elaborated below.

Much of the scholarship on global care chains focuses on micro-processes rather than on analyzing how these fit into a global political economy of care (there are important exceptions: Parreñas 2001a; Kofman and Raghuram 2007; Lutz 2008; Yeates 2009) and what the normative implications might be for global justice. This chapter aims to create some pathways for thinking about and linking these analytical and normative issues. The following section identifies the dimensions of an analysis of a transnational political economy of care in which the specific practices associated with the employment of migrant women working in home-based domestic or care work find themselves. The term "transnational" (as opposed to "global") is used here to denote the significance of the meso/macro relationship – that is, of the political, economic, and social relationships that belong to and connect differently situated national and supranational states. The final part of the chapter uses the ethics of care as an analytical method and normative guide to explore the implications for global justice of this transnational political economy of care.

There are a number of reasons why developing a wider analysis of the increase in transnational home-based care provision may be helpful. In a context in which women globally are taking on more responsibilities to earn income without a significant reduction of their care responsibilities, the transnational movement of women into care and domestic work in private households represents a profoundly asymmetrical solution – not only between women and men but also between poorer and richer regions – to women's attempts to reconcile these dual responsibilities. For migrant workers, crossing continents to earn money provides an important opportunity, but it is also an opportunity that involves entering a world in which migration rules ensure that they have different (and limited) rights to social, economic, political, and intimate citizenship than do their employers. Furthermore, these limitations give rise to the likelihood that women will enter the often unregulated world of domestic and care work in the home.

The conditions of this work perpetuate two forms of inequality: (1) the devaluation and invisibility of the private-care domain and its subservience to the public world of work and (2) the translation of the unequal relations of personal interdependency into the unequal relations of transnational interdependency.

This raises important questions not only about the rights of migrants but also about work/life reconciliation policies, about how gender equality is framed and understood by policy makers, and about global inequalities in the provision of and need for care. These dynamics, and the need for global strategies to mitigate them, become more apparent when one understands them as part of a broader transnational political economy of care. In its turn, this demands a normative approach to global justice informed by an understanding of the centrality of care in everyday life. It is to the first of these that I now turn.

Dimensions of a Transnational Political Economy of Care

Following on from an attempt to understand how social welfare policies (for care, employment, work/care balance) influence the demand and provision for home-based domestic and care workers, my concern is with how European nation-welfare-states exist within a situation of unequal geopolitical interdependence. I propose that transnational home-based care provision be understood as part of a transnational political economy of care and that this involves a number of different but synchronic dimensions: (1) the movement of care labour; (2) the dynamics of care commitments; (3) the movement of care capital; (4) the influence of care discourses and policies; and (5) the development of social movements, non-governmental organizations (NGOs), and grassroots organizations.

First, the migration of women from poorer to richer regions into home-based care work is part of a wider process – the transnational movement of care labour. The relationship between migration, gender, and care also involves professional and semi-professional health, social work, education, and care workers working in small and large state, religious, independent, and private-sector institutions (Kofman, Raghuram, and Merefield 2005; Yeates 2004a; Yeates 2009). Indeed, the notion of the global care chain itself tends to generalize what is only one type of migrant worker (a mother who has left her children in her country of origin in the global South to find work in the global North looking after the children of her employer). The situation of migrant care workers is typically very diverse and, as far as home-based domestic and care work are concerned, transnational connections also operate *within* regions of both the global North and the global South. Thus, for example, domestic workers from Malaysia go to Indonesia while Indonesian women find work in Singapore and in Saudi Arabia, which also provides work for women from the Philippines and Sri Lanka. Within the North, enlargement of the European Union since 2004 has seen an increase in highly educated young women migrants from Central and Eastern Europe finding care and domestic work in Northern, Western, and Southern Europe, often as a stepping stone to more professional work. These migration trails transect tracks of old colonial relations (e.g., Ethiopians to Italy, Indian and African workers to the United Kingdom, and South American workers to Spain) as well as ties of religion (e.g., Roman Catholicism connects the Philippines with Italy and Spain) (Piper 2003; Kofman and Raghuram 2007; Lutz 2008). In addition, the conditions of domestic and care work in the home take many different forms: employees may provide housework or child care or both; they may live in or live out; they may work a few hours a week, a few hours a day, or full time (often very long hours); their work may involve acting as a carer or cleaner for an older, frail person or a disabled person, or it may involve being their personal assistant, inside and outside the house. An employee may be self-employed, "undeclared" (receiving cash-in-hand as part of the grey economy), or may work for a private agency or for a local authority. As migrant workers, they may be working under a special permit (say, as an "au pair") or they may be undocumented. Not all migrant workers leave their children in their country of origin: in Spain, for example, migrants are likely to bring not only their children but also their mothers (to provide child care while they work). Not all women migrants in care work have children, and in some countries this work is also done by men.

These home-based workers are less numerically significant in the international division of reproductive labour, however, than are formal health and care workers. In 2000, in the United Kingdom, the international recruitment of nurses, teachers, and doctors meant that 31 percent of doctors and 13 percent of nurses were non-UK born; in London, this was 23 percent and 47 percent, respectively (Glover et al. 2001). Half of those workers contributing to the expansion of the UK National Health Service in the early 2000s had qualified abroad. By the end of 2005, 30 percent of its doctors and 10 percent of its nurses had received their initial training overseas (Crisp 2007, 16). Recruitment to teaching is also high: one recruitment agency in London said that, without migrant teachers, London schools would fall apart (Glover et al. 2001, 37). In France, a quarter of all hospital doctors are foreign or naturalized; in Germany, nurses are recruited from Eastern Europe; in Norway, from Poland (Kofman et al. 2000; Bach 2003). What is also significant is the active role states play in recruiting health personnel, especially, but not only, to the United States, Canada, and the United Kingdom. Furthermore, the growth of private agencies working for the private health sector has also marked recent developments (Bach 2003). In the United Kingdom, campaigns aimed at nurses from India and the Philippines have recruited them into both the health service and private-sector nursing (RCN 2002). According to Adversario (2003), each year over 70 percent of the seven thousand Filipina nurses who graduate will emigrate (cited in Bach 2003, 4), partly encouraged by policies of the former Marcos regime, which saw emigration and the receipt of foreign exchange through remittances as part of its development strategy. While this has kept private-sector agencies in business, the Philippine Nursing Association has been more concerned with its effect on the health-care infrastructure (Yeates 2009, 86).

Building on Parreñas's work, Yeates (2009) seeks to widen the concept of global care chains by identifying further types of chains that operate within a "new international division of reproductive labour": global nursing care chains and global religious care chains. The latter refer to vocational religious workers who travel abroad to provide care work through non-governmental, religious, charitable, and voluntary-sector organizations. This serves to highlight the diversity of care work, its transnational hierarchies, and the numerous forms of agencies operating in tandem with the state at a transnational level.[2] In relation to the hierarchy of nursing chains, Yeates observes:

> Countries at the top of the chain are "fed" by those lower down the ranks: for example, the United States draws nurses from Canada; Canada draws nurses from England to make up for its losses to the United States; England draws from South Africa to fill its vacancies; South Africa draws on Swaziland. Countries at the bottom end of the nursing chain may supply international markets but not replenish their stocks by importing health workers from other countries: the Philippines is a major example of this. The problem for such countries is that they have no further countries from which they may recruit to make up for the losses of their own nurses (80).

Health professionals, especially those from developing countries, share commonalities in their working lives with migrant home-based care workers:

gender and racial discrimination, lack of recognition of skills and qualifications in pay levels, concentration in the least desirable areas of specialization. Migrant workers may pay into national insurance systems but not be eligible for benefits while, at the same time, missing out in contributions to insurance systems in their own countries (Bach 2003; Kofman, Ragurham, and Merefield 2005).

Together, through their labour, home-based and professional migrant care workers serve to reduce the social expenditure costs of the countries in which they work. The rising costs of child care and elder care created by an aging society and women's increased participation in paid work is relieved by the employment of low-paid care workers, and the rising costs of health care are held back by the recruitment of lower-paid health workers whose training costs have been met by poorer countries. This constitutes a double whammy for the migrants' countries of origin. It increases the care deficit through the absence of formal and informal carers and it strips the health and care systems in those countries of their vital resources. The transnational transfers of skill and caring resources constitute a major form of geo-political inequality. Moreover, in those areas such as Africa, where health-care needs have been exacerbated by poverty and AIDS, it has precipitated a health and care crisis (Bach 2003). While recognizing the push factors involved in professional migration in his overview of the migration of health workers, Bach (2003, ix) nevertheless comments: "It is an indictment of governments and employers that they prefer to rely on the relatively straightforward panacea of international recruitment rather than focusing on underlying problems of pay and working conditions."

It would be wrong to assume that this phenomenon is new. Some of the developments we see now are the result not only of globalization but also of historical precedents, especially colonialism and postcolonialism. From the early twentieth century, the welfare gains of the working class were presented by British governments as the fruits of imperialism (Williams 1989). Later in Britain, in the 1950s and 1960s, the recruitment of health and care labour from the colonies both provided cheap labour for the new institutions of the welfare state and met a labour shortage that otherwise would have had to have been filled by married women, thus preventing the disruption of the normative practice of the male breadwinner society, in which women are assumed to have primary responsibilities to the home and children. Similar strategies were followed later in Germany and Switzerland, where guest workers were brought in. In the 1960s, Sweden, with a different gender, migration, and labour history from Britain and Germany, opted to recruit women rather than migrants into the labour market. This is not the whole story, for these migrant workers were often pathologized and marginalized in Europe. In Britain, nurses and cleaners from the Caribbean were vilified as working mothers. They may have been allowed to build the postwar welfare states, but they were not always deemed eligible to receive state services (Williams 1989, 1995). Compare that with today, when the use of migrant domestic and care labour prevents the disruption of the new adult worker model of welfare, in which women are encouraged to engage in paid employment. Then and today, these were seen as cost-effective ways of securing family norms and meeting care needs (even though these norms and needs have now changed). Then and today, these women's social relations and citizenship rights were inscribed with gendered and racialized inequalities.

In the last decade, some recruiting countries have begun to acknowledge some responsibility, and trade unions have moved away from a position of protecting indigenous workers towards setting up mentoring programs for migrant workers, zero-tolerance strategies on racism, and so on. Nevertheless, the home as workplace is often exempt from anti-discriminatory policies and social protection, although moves in Spain to regularize domestic work have involved the trade unions. In 2003, Sweden committed all its ministries to examine how they could contribute to more just development policies (Deacon 2007, 181-82). In the United Kingdom, the Department of Health acknowledged its role as a global employer of health workers. By 2006, it claimed to be the only developed country to have an ethical recruitment code that applies to both the National Health Service and private employers with regard to preventing them from "poaching" health-care workers from countries in Sub-Saharan Africa. This includes providing training and support (e.g., topping up doctors' wages) to encourage health workers to work in their countries of origin as well as a commitment to press EU member states to take similar action (DfID 2006). At the same time, reliance on overseas recruitment continues, often exercised through private agencies that are harder to bring into line. Bach (2003) suggests that bilateral agreements between countries over recruitment work better than national codes of practice: they circumvent the need for private agencies; they are more transparent, and they can be used innovatively to support training and induction as well as the temporary payment of health workers' salaries in their countries of origin when they return.

The second dimension of the transnational political economy of care is the transnational dynamics of care commitments as people move to different countries and leave behind younger or older people to be cared for at a distance, or, in their turn, have no family locally to care for their needs (Baldock 2000; Parreñas 2001a; Ackers and Stalford 2004; Pyle 2006). Usually children are left in the care of other female relatives, thus reinforcing care as women's responsibility.[3] While family separation through migration is not new, its widespread experience through regional and global migration is. As far as migrant care workers are concerned, research shows that maintaining family commitments and intimate connections over long temporal and spatial distances is an extremely important and inventive aspect of life. The concept of the "economic" migrant tends to displace the significance of diasporic affective ties. Care workers from Central Europe who work in the grey economy looking after older people in Austria organize two weekly shifts by family members to ensure continuity back home (Österle and Hammer 2007). Parreñas (2001a) shows that migrant mothers develop complex strategies in constrained circumstances (long work hours, costs of travel, etc.) to maintain communication with their children. She also shows that families are adaptive to separation but, at the same time, that this separation creates pain and longing on both sides. Migrant care workers' needs for work/care balance are both less supported and more precipitous than are those of the women for whom they are working. As with the history of migrant women workers (see, for example, Reynolds [2005] on Caribbean mothers in the United Kingdom), it is not that migrating women simply become earners but that their concept of good motherhood absorbs the identity of provider.

Migrant workers and their families' care needs challenge nation-based eligibility for care support services, financial supports for caring, pension entitlements, and provisions for flexibility of care responsibilities at work (e.g., when these may require someone to cross continents to care for a dying parent). These care needs are often exacerbated by migration rules that proscribe entry to particular categories of family member (e.g., children above a certain age, elderly parents). In the United Arab Emirates, parents can apply for child reunion only when they have income above a certain level (Kofman and Rhaguram 2007, 15).

The disproportionate amount of care responsibilities across the globe needs to be put into this picture. While the richer areas of the North are concerned with a "care deficit" consequent upon women's employment and an aging population, the developing world is experiencing a crisis of care as AIDS, chronic illness, and/or natural disasters place enormous burdens on women who are expected to do the caring with very little infrastructural support. Thus, earning for women takes the form of home-based piecework, domestic work, and working in family businesses. These jobs are usually lacking in social protection and in rights to organize and, unlike the part-time work that women in the North engage in outside the home, are carried on *in parallel* to care and domestic responsibilities (Hassim 2006). Indeed, women have found themselves taking on new responsibilities, such as debt repayment (Beneria and Floro 2006, 212). Work and care responsibilities are particularly onerous and have expanded with increases in divorce, lone parenting, and the care needs associated with HIV/AIDS; yet, they still remain invisible in development strategies that focus on men's paid employment.

Associated with this is the movement of wages and the remittances that migrant workers send home, which need to be seen as part of the material care provided for family members. The subject of remittances is too big to rehearse here; suffice it to say that they contain contradictory consequences. On the one hand, they may provide women migrants with agency and, in aggregate, constitute a major cushioning against poverty for developing countries: they total twice the overseas aid that goes to poorer countries (Brown 2006, 58). On the other hand, they also create significant hardship for those who send them (Datta et al. 2007) and are often highly individualized rather than collective in the way they are spent. Women's remittances are particularly important as sources of support for the costs of care, education, and health, especially if they are not only sent but also received by women (Orozco, Lowell, and Schneider 2006).[4] Kofman and Rhaguram (2007) note that they may also constitute forms of remuneration for caring activities carried out by relatives. In this way, remittances reveal double forms of geo-political exploitation that are further exemplified, as Yeates (2009, 120) notes, by the fact that those from migrant nurses often go to fund the training of the next generation of nurses. Remittances also usually involve brokers or financial institutions, and these form an important part of the meso level of institutional support.

The third dimension of the transnational political economy of care is the transnational movement of care capital. Trends towards the commodification of care provision have accelerated the intervention of the private market in health and social care. Market competition has led to the dominance of large international organizations (Holden 2002). This has intensified with the nation-state's contracting out to private cleaning, catering, and refuse collection companies. And, increasingly, these are located outside the nation-state within which they operate. Holden (2002) gives examples of corporations that have expanded into long-term care in the United Kingdom.

The British United Provident Association developed operations in Spain, Ireland, Thailand, Hong Kong, and Saudi Arabia, while Ashbourne, the second largest provider of long-term elder care in the United Kingdom in the early 2000s, was owned by the American Sun Healthcare, which also holds subsidiaries in Spain, Australia, and Germany. Because of the labour-intensive nature of care, profits are made through economies of scale, often forcing the smaller more specialist provider out of the market. Efficiency strategies pursued by large corporations (such as deskilling) often influence those developed in the state sector. Quality of care is ceded in favour of greater standardization, making these providers "market-following" rather than "client-seeking" (Holden 2002, 62). Another area of expansion involves recruitment agencies for care work (especially nursing), which operate under varying degrees of regulation (Bach 2003; Yeates 2009).

Brennan's (2007) forensic study of the corporation ABC Learning describes how child care became big business in Australia. Government subsidies to the organization made massive profits possible. In 2006, ABC expanded into the United States, and, in 2007, one of the biggest providers of private nursery care in the United Kingdom, Nord Anglia, agreed to sell its nurseries to ABC Learning for £31.2 million, making ABC the biggest child-care chain in the United Kingdom (Boone 2007; Brennan 2007, 217). When ABC was hit by the credit crunch in 2007, it was subsequently bailed out by the Australian government in 2008 with $(Aus)22 million.[5] By 2009, the company was looking to sell over seven hundred of its child-care centres. These examples demonstrate how, because care work lacks the potential for increasing profit through increasing productivity, the principles of market investment (risk, expansion, profit) conflict with the principles of care provision (individual needs, continuity, and quality service provided by skilled labour). Collective commitment to public subsidy does not guarantee quality and equity, but it provides a sounder basis from which to meet them.

The fourth dimension of the transnational political economy of care involves the transnational influence of care discourses and policies.[6] Reference has already been made to the convergence in ways of delivering care services in Europe, influenced in part by the European Union's policies as well as by cross-national models within EU member states. The commodification of care and the related discourse of "choice" for service use, which accompanied the introduction of forms of cash or tax allowances, is one such example. The "spread" across Europe of paternity leave is another (Lister et al. 2007).

Perhaps the best illustration of transnational influence in the area of care is the way "social investment" has become a dominant discourse underpinning the implementation of work/care reconciliation policies in the European Union, international organizations, and national governments (Dobrowolsky and Jenson 2004; Jenson 2008; Jenson and Saint-Martin 2006; Mahon 2010a). Its key characteristic is investment in the capabilities of human capital – mothers as workers and children as citizen-workers-of-the-future. This is to be achieved through supports for labour market activation, anti-poverty measures, education, and child care through services that represent good value for money, with the aim of maintaining competitiveness in the global economy. These ideas have been developed by the OECD (2006), which, in *Starting Strong*, argues the need to invest in early childhood programs, and its influence can be seen in UNESCO and UNICEF policies (Mahon 2010a). Jenson (2008) points out the overlap in the OECD and the Economic Commission for Latin America and the Caribbean (ECLAC 2007), and Molyneux's (2006) account of *Progresa/Oportunidades* programs developed since 1997 in Mexico shows how anti-poverty policies are framed in terms of the need to develop human capital. The problems in this program illustrate general difficulties with the social investment approach. While highlighting women's care responsibilities, it sidesteps crucial issues of women's empowerment by ignoring women's voice and gender inequalities in the division of household labour. The recognition of care involves more than an investment in women's maternal roles: it requires challenging the structural inequalities that underpin its practice and the subservience of its policies to economic development. Collective voices that can articulate such challenges are also important, and it is to these that I now turn.

The fifth dimension of the transnational political economy of care – the development of transnational social movements, NGOs, and grassroots organizations – characterizes recent political activity. In relation to care activism, while care policy making is dominated in Europe by the ideas of social investment, social movements and NGOs have tended to organize around social justice – the recognition of care needs and responsibilities and their redistribution (Williams 2009). Women's movements also have a long tradition of organizing and have been influential in generating global women's conferences such as that in Beijing in 1995 (Mayo 2005). Similarly, within Europe, the European Women's Lobby (EWL) organizes for women's interests to be present and recognized within EU debates (Hoskyns 1996). Ensuring that women's organizations represent the interests of minority women and migrants, and that migrant organizations represent the interests of migrant women, has been tricky (Williams 2003). Yet, the EWL has recently taken up two key themes: care and migrant women (EWL 2007).

The latter emerged from the 1990s work of the Black and Migrants Women's Group, which drew together experiences from migrant women's associations across Europe to highlight issues around domestic and care work (EWL 1995; Williams 2003). The EWL argues for improvements in public services and attention to the rights of female migrant care and domestic workers, citing the activity of the European Trade Union Confederation in recognizing people's needs for domestic help while ensuring adequate protection, conditions, and remuneration for those who are employed in such work.[7] In the United Kingdom, the organization *Kalayaan* works for migrant domestic and care workers both nationally and transnationally (Oxfam and Kalayaan 2008).

Disability movements have also organized transnationally, especially in taking up disability as a social development and human rights issue.[8] According to the UN Development Programme, 80 percent of disabled people live in developing countries, account for 15 to 20 percent of the world's poorest, and are often not included in rural poverty alleviation programs (Action on Disability and Development 2009). The UN Convention on the Rights of Persons with Disabilities focuses on respect, autonomy, and independence; on freedom from discrimination; on inclusion, participation, and equality. In relation to carers, in 2007, the organization Eurocarers was established to represent the voice of informal carers and to pressure for change across Europe and within the European Union. Lobbying by networks of activists and researchers is also common in this area as in others – such as the influence of the European Commission Childcare Network in the EU commission's 1992 Recommendation on Childcare.

Some of these campaigns and activities have percolated upwards to the global arena. For example, the International Labour Organization (ILO) has sought to protect workers worldwide through its core labour standards, and the UN has sought to protect the human rights of migrant workers. The 2006 *Report of the Global Commission on International Migration* recommends increased international cooperation and agreements between states to secure the rights to social security and health care of migrant workers (Deacon 2007, 161-62). Nevertheless, the extent to which the issues of care needs and responsibilities have been taken on board at this level is a different matter.

Global Justice and the Political Ethics of Care

While the policy processes of global governance are sometimes informed by gender, policy discussions, critiques, and conclusions tend to decentre some of the issues that are key to gender equality, such as care of older and disabled people (and the rights of those people themselves), child-care provision, and the forms of social protection that provide rights to give and to receive care. In terms of the former, the World Bank (2002) has now taken on board gender mainstreaming. Yet, its statement on social policy made at the end of 2005 (the "Arusha Statement")[9] – tide-turning as it seemed to be in its focus upon citizens' rights, an accountable state, welfare funded from taxation, and empowerment of the poor – made no mention of gender relations in general or care in particular. Where the World Bank does mention these, as in the *World Development Report 2006*, it talks about the economic investment that children represent. Yet, as Razavi (2007, 30-31) comments, the World Bank is "silent about the huge amount of unpaid care work that goes on in all societies to sustain infants and children (as well as people who are elderly, sick or disabled, and also able-bodied adults) on a day-to-day basis and from one generation to the next."[10] A similar elision occurs in writing on international relations, migration, and global social policy.[11] Deacon's (2007, 169-93) normative conclusions on the future of global governance, for example, importantly identify how women have brought pressure to bear on international organizations. Yet, it is not clear what this implies for ideas on global justice. For this, we need to turn to those whose approach to global social justice embeds, theoretically and empirically, everyday social relations of care within macro understandings of inequality (e.g., Tronto 1993; Robinson 2006a, 2006b; Held 2005; Hankivsky 2004, 2006).

The ethics of care is useful both as a method of analysis and as a normative framework. As a method, the ethics of care emphasizes the *interdependence* of individuals and the embeddedness of their thinking and acting in social relations rather than in autonomous rational action (Hankivsky 2004).[12] It also presupposes that human flourishing is the key to our sustainability and, therefore, that the conditions for this – care and cooperation – are central. Second, the ethics of care demands our being *sensitive to context* as opposed to assuming universals and assessing them through impartial reason. This alerts us to the complexity of power mediated through class, ethnicity, gender, and other social relations. The third element of a care ethics is *responsiveness,* an ability to perceive others on their own terms, emphasizing the need for the marginalized to have access to conditions that enable them to articulate their needs. Finally, these ethics alert us to the *consequences of choices:* What are the material and practical outcomes of actions on people's lives? How do we ensure that people may give and receive care?

We can apply this analysis to the transnational political economy of care. The emphasis on interdependence can refer not only to individuals but also to nation-states: just as the male breadwinner was constructed as independent and his wife as dependent, and feminists revealed how his autonomy was actually dependent on the hidden care and support of his wife, so we could say a similar thing about nation-welfare-states. The capacity to meet the care needs of their welfare subjects is partly the outcome of global interdependencies. This has the consequence of intensifying the difficulties of meeting the care needs of the poorer regions. It is therefore incumbent upon any notion of global justice to think of these care needs as well as those of the West.

This analysis implies a concern with the transnational consequences of state actions. When developed states cut the wage costs of care workers, the consequence is labour shortages whose short-term solution is international recruitment of cheaper labour, which, in its turn, results in care deficits in poorer regions. Similarly, where work/care balance policies in developed countries are underpinned by the primary aims of encouraging women into the workforce and developing cost-effective care services, and where gender equality at home and at work remains secondary, seeking work/care balance for caregivers becomes an individual responsibility often met through other women's labour. When that labour is migrant labour, it may entail major work/care imbalances for the worker as well as care deficits in her country of origin. This means we should adopt an expansive and transnational understanding of gender equality and of work/care balance.

Kofman and Rhaguram (2007, 12) suggest that, in this situation, we need to be aware of four sets of care relations: the migrant workers who provide care; the care responsibilities for those whom the worker has left behind; the responsibilities of those who the worker brings with her; and a migrant's own care needs, now or in the future. Such an approach highlights a contextual sensitivity to the different ways in which women and men in the North and the South are attempting to reconcile their work/care responsibilities in the context of globalization. An ethics of care further demands an awareness of the challenges that exist for developing countries with regard to integrating care priorities into institutional policies. Here, the dominant productivist logic is not always tempered by a social investment approach (as it is in a number of developed welfare societies) and, thus, aggressively situates social development as secondary to economic development, creating difficulties for prioritizing care policies. There are also limits to the "dual earner/carer" model of family life. In many developing countries, the earning and caring configurations within families are complex, diverse, and multiple, situated in conditions in which responsibilities attach to broad kin networks, where pooling of income is widespread, and where members may need to migrate to earn (Hassim 2006). Where informal employment is commonplace for women, an insurance system tied to employment is less favourable to women than are universal benefits funded through the tax system. Fundamentally, women's political voice is crucial. What global North and global South share, however, is the need to reshape ideas of global justice not simply to include more explicit care policies but also to reframe these with reference to the practices and ethics of interdependence, contextual sensitivity, responsiveness, and responsibility for the consequence of choice.

Robinson (2006a, 2006b) argues that, while social protection standards, employment rights, and human rights through international organizations are essential, they are not, in the long run, enough. For example, she does not deny the importance of the ILO's core labour standards as hooks for claims to, say, the rights to collective bargaining or the protection of children. Nevertheless, she argues that such standards are based on the rights-holder as an atomized individual rather than as an individual constituted through her/his relations of care/support for and from others. This being the case, these rights do not really begin to challenge the thinking that situates social questions of care as subordinate to economic issues of productivity, profit, and performance. According to Robinson, it would be far better if we could embed rights within the knowledge that all people need to care and to be cared for.

Conclusion

The relationship between migration and care needs to be understood as part of the transnational dynamics of the political economy of care. Care labour, work/care balance, and care commitments must be seen as transnational issues requiring transnational and global strategies. We need to enlarge the conception of global social justice so that it encompasses the everyday reality of care in people's lives as it occurs within transnational processes of migration and globalization. These transnational processes are not simply the consequence of contemporary globalization: they are also the consequence of colonialism and its links to nation-welfare-state building. With regard to developing a theoretical framework for understanding the relationship between migration, care, and welfare states, I propose that we need different levels of analysis (micro, meso, and macro) in order to link individual care practices in different countries to social, cultural, and policy discourses and contexts at local, national, regional, and global levels.

From the perspective of the developed world, the notion of work/care balance is limited: it presupposes lives that are centred on the private sphere of the family, the contained area of work, and the contained space of territorial citizenship. It seems to have little space for the social, the civil, or the creative. It has no place for creative ventures, for community-based or voluntary activities, or for those practices (often driven by an ethic of interdependence or mutuality) that contribute to a flourishing civil society. It requires an enlarged and imaginative understanding of what "work" is, what "care" is, and where the geographic limits of care and work are situated.

People not only need time and capacity to ensure they can support and care for themselves and close others but also the time and capacity to care for the "world" in the sense of a wider community that is both local and global. This is where a political ethics of care is relevant to recognizing an interdependence that is wider than family, more encompassing than the productivist ethic of work, and more spatially complex than the local, private household, while, at the same time, being part of our understanding of what it means to be a global citizen.

2

Migration and Globalized Care Work
The Case of Internationally Educated Nurses in Canada

CHRISTINA GABRIEL

The feminization of migration has prompted feminists to consider the dimensions and consequences of transnational care work. To date, much feminist scholarship has been directed at the care labour done by migrant women workers, specifically those activities constructed as "low-skilled," such as working as a nanny or cleaner. Yet, care labour also encompasses migrant women's work in the "skilled" sectors, such as nursing and teaching.[1] Throughout the global economic North, countries are experiencing nursing shortages, and Canada is no exception. It is estimated that the country will experience a shortfall of some 113,000 registered nurses by 2016 (RNAO 2008, 8). Within this context, the movement of Internationally Educated Nurses (IENs) across borders is an increasingly important aspect of the transnationalization of care work.[2] This chapter focuses on the role of the Canadian state in the transfer of nursing labour and demonstrates that this trend is not straightforward. The terms that govern the entry of IENs to Canada are framed by an array of permanent and temporary immigration categories that result in differential access to the rights and benefits associated with citizenship. These terms are further complicated by the rules that regulate entry to the registered nurse occupation. Taken together, these two aspects of governance play a critical role in determining whether IENs are actually able to work as nurses in Canada, despite the ongoing shortage.

This discussion situates the case of IENs within a conceptual framework that draws on feminist scholarship on migration, social reproduction, and hierarchal citizenship. It then briefly considers the relationship between the nursing shortages and neoliberalism. The final portion of the chapter examines how the immigration regime and process of credentialing is implicated in the construction and recognition of "skilled" caring labour. Here, the experiences of IENs in Canada contradict the widely held neoliberal tenet that skilled migrants can circulate freely, without impediment, throughout the global economy.

Gender, Globalized Care Work, and Hierarchal Citizenship

Processes of globalization have prompted states in both the global economic North and South to engage in various rounds of neoliberal-inspired state strategies, including privatization, welfare state cuts, and public-sector retrenchment, which have contributed to a restructuring of care. Feminist scholars have traced how the changing provision of care has increased women's community and household responsibilities at both the local and the national scales. The restructuring of care also has a transnational dimension, as growing numbers of migrant women workers cross borders to engage in various forms of care work. This section illustrates how the changing dynamics of social reproduction, globalized care work, and citizenship frame the migration of skilled migrant care workers.

Feminists have been at the fore of analyzing the consequences of neoliberal restructuring and processes of globalization on social reproduction and its governance (Bakker and Silvey 2008; Bezanson and Luxton 2006). Indeed, social reproduction has been a central, albeit contested, concept within feminist political economy. Bezanson and Luxton (2006, 3) provide a concise definition: "Social reproduction refers to the processes involved in maintaining and reproducing people, specifically the labouring population, and their labour power on a daily and generational basis." Following Yeates (2009, 5), care is considered a particular form of social reproductive labour, one that refers to a host of tasks that support and sustain "people as physical, social and cultural beings." This conception of social reproduction and care brings into focus a complex set of relations and activities – from women's unpaid work in the home to women's paid participation in state-provided and private health, welfare, and education sectors.

The division between a masculinized public realm and a feminized private realm, and the concomitant devaluing of tasks and values associated with the latter, structures the gendered nature of care work. Here, a particular set of understandings comes into play, most notably that it is women who "have a natural capacity and desire to provide care" and, as a result, that it is primarily women who should shoulder the responsibility for paid and unpaid care work (Meyer 2000, 6). The provision of care ranges from formalized types of care, including health and social care associated with particular welfare regimes, to more informalized forms of care (Kofman and Raghuram 2009, iii). Registered nursing, a profession dominated overwhelmingly by women, is an important example of formalized care work. Whereas much care work is constructed as "unskilled" and, therefore, undervalued, nursing, in contrast, offers an example of an occupation that is widely regarded as "skilled." Registered nurses are required to have postsecondary educations and to complete a set of training competencies that place them within a category of "skilled" occupations. As McNeil-Walsh (2008, 143) notes: "The very nature of nursing, a profession which embodies a 'duty to care' means that those skills are valued on a societal level and considered to be crucial to a society's well being and ability to operate effectively."

Nevertheless, economic downturns in the 1980s and 1990s resulted in widespread cuts to health budgets, and the nursing workforce was a major target. This restructuring was a major contributor to a nursing shortage in the global economic North (Kingma 2006, 29-30). The increasing shortage of registered nurses in many countries can be considered an instantiation of what Zimmerman, Litt, and Bose (2006, 10) term a "crisis of care," referring to "the ongoing and serious changes in our social systems of caring that have been wrought by globalization."

On a national scale, states can address critical nursing shortages by improving the domestic labour supply through developments in education and training and through the pursuit of retention strategies, including improvements to wages and working conditions. Alternatively, international recruitment on a transnational scale can be deployed to address the crisis of care. Figures indicate that "foreign trained nurses accounted for 23% of the nurse workforce in New Zealand in 2002; 6% in Canada (2001); 8% in Ireland (2002) and the UK (2001); and 4% in the United States (2000)" (Batata 2005, 1). To the extent that countries use migration policy to manage their deficits in care, these figures will only increase. Many IENs come from the global economic South. Legacies of colonialism that resulted in the unequal positioning of countries within a global order, and the impact of more recent neoliberal structural adjustment programs, create a set of circumstances that prompt nurses to immigrate to more developed countries (Stasiulis and Bakan 2003; United Nations Population Fund 2006, 27). In some cases, such as the Philippines, states themselves are implicated in a strategy that explicitly produces nurses for employment abroad (Ball 2008;

Onuki this volume). The movement of IENs can also take place regionally within the global economic North. For example, there is considerable nurse migration from Canada to the United States (Gabriel 2008). Canada, like Australia and the United Kingdom, both imports and exports nurse labour (Yeates 2009, 79). Migration becomes a survival strategy for some and/or a means of professional enhancement for others.

The global movement of women across borders has been characterized as the "feminization of migration" (UNFPA 2006, 23), a description that nicely captures the increasing importance of women's mobility by drawing attention to the numbers – "nearly half (49.6 per cent) of all international migrants are women" (21). At the same time, attention is focused on how gendered assumptions and norms underwrite the differing migration experiences of men and women. As Nicola Piper (2006, 139) writes: "Policies affect men and women differently for three principal reasons: the concentration of men and women in different migratory flows based on gender-segregated labor markets 'at home' and abroad; gendered socio-economic power structures; and sociocultural definitions of appropriate roles in destination as well as origin countries." Increasingly, feminist scholars have been concerned to demonstrate not only the ways in which care work is implicated in cross-border mobility but also which groups of women are engaged in this activity (Ehrenreich and Hochschild 2002; Hondagneu-Sotelo 2000; Parreñas 2001a, 2005b; Pratt 2004). In an effort to explore the connections between transnational migration, gender, and care, Arlie Hochschild (2000, 131) conceptualizes a *global care chain* to characterize "a series of personal links between people across the globe based on the paid or unpaid work of caring." Yeates acknowledges the merits of this formulation but makes an important intervention when she argues for a broader understanding of the global care chain. In her view, the concept of a global care chain would, first, recognize the importance of skilled migrant care workers; second, move beyond an exclusive focus on mothers with children to consider a broader range of kinship ties; and, finally, emphasize other forms of care, such as health, education, sexual, and religious as well as taking into account the experiences of care workers in different sectors (Yeates 2009, 50-53). According to Yeates, the transfer of care can be interrogated using an expanded version of the global care chain that embraces three analytic elements: inputs and outputs, such as education, training, and recruitment; territoriality; and the internal and external relations of governance (59). In so doing, she expands the concept of a "global care chain" to include other types of care chains.

The global migration of registered nurses offers an exemplar of skilled migrant care work (Yeates 2004a, 2009; Ball 2004). Indeed, as Kofman and Raghuram argue, an examination of how skilled women migrants are positioned within reproductive labour is crucial for a number of reasons. First, skilled women migrants are active participants in social reproduction organized by the state; second, migrant women make an important contribution as providers of welfare, in contrast to dominant perceptions that cast them as clients and receivers of welfare; and, third, migrants are selected differentially by national migration regimes: "It appears that skilled women migrants are being enticed to migrate precisely in order to provide welfare" (Kofman and Raghuram 2006, 283). Thus, analyzing gender and global labour markets forces a reconsideration of the way in which social reproduction is multiply sited, but it also necessitates consideration of the ways in which it is being restructured globally (297). As the work of Yeates (2009) and Kofman and Raghuram (2006, 2009) underscores, if we are to understand the complex dimensions and contradictions of the transfer of care across borders, it is necessary to consider all the sectors in which care work takes place as well as the different levels of skills required.

Yeates's formulation of a global care chain contains a number of elements. Although it is beyond the scope of this chapter to examine each of these in turn, her understanding of "governance" in relation to nursing care chains is critical to this analysis. For Yeates (2009, 61), "the focus of governance lies with the regulation of care labour together with the regulation (however minimal it may be) of care provision itself. The former pertains to the entry of labour into the destination country and the care sector, while the latter relates to the working conditions and delivery of the service itself."

States emerge as powerful actors in so far as they play a role in facilitating or barring the entry of different kinds of migrant workers through the construction of complex national immigration regimes. The migration of care workers thus raises broader normative and policy questions about the nature of citizenship and rights.

As Bosniak (2009, 135) argues, the increasing transnationalization of care forces a consideration of citizenship practice centred not on the familiar discursive terrain of inclusion and belonging but, rather, on boundaries, exclusivity, and closure: "Here, citizenship is concerned with the community's threshold — with the boundaries of that community in the first instance. This citizenship is a status that assigns persons to membership in specific political communities — ordinarily, nation states. And the status of citizenship in any given nation is almost always restricted." This understanding of citizenship foregrounds the way citizenship is implicated in processes of differentiation and stratification.

Citizenship as a status bestows membership in a nation-state, but nation-states themselves are positioned in a set of unequal relations of power. Stephen Castles (2005, 210-11) traces the emergence of a new global order following the end of the Cold War, one founded on a "hierarchical nation-state system." While nation-states in the international system are constructed as equal in formal legal terms, geo-political realities demonstrate that "power flows from the centre through a number of intermediate level states, to be imposed on the weakest countries of the South" (213), as is reflected in the workings of international law and trade. The differential positioning of nation-states in terms of political, military, economic, and cultural capacity leads to a similar hierarchy of rights and freedoms of their peoples, or, as Castles puts it, "hierarchical citizenship" (215).

This dynamic of inequality finds expression in the reorganization of reproductive labour on a global scale, where women migrants, frequently from the global South, provide various forms of care work for women-citizen-employers in the North (Stasiulis and Bakan 2003; Maher 2004; Parreñas 2001b). In an effort to capture the contradictory citizenship positions that low-wage migrant care workers occupy within host countries, Parreñas (2001b, 1134) alludes to a state of "partial citizenship," whereby the political, civil, and social incorporation of low-wage migrants in host societies is restricted. One of the mechanisms that produces partial citizenship is border control — associated with the migration regime — that acts as a "flexible filter" (Anderson and Shuttleworth 2004, 153) through which migrants are differentially incorporated.

In this respect, Castles (2005, 219) and others have also recognized how the migration policies of states themselves produce various forms of internal stratification (Kofman 2008). As Stasiulis and Bakan (2003, 11) put it:

> [The] selective criminalization of certain types of migrants and the privileged treatment of others in migration processes and policies create and reinforce the hierarchal nature of national citizenship. They affect which migrants are treated as "fit" candidates for host-society citizenship, which enter with probationary status and can be "re-fitted" at their own expense, and which are rendered completely ineligible.

The terms that govern a migrant worker's mode of entry to a national community produce a number of statuses, including citizens, naturalized citizens, permanent residents, temporary workers, foreign students, tourists, refugees, and those without status. Thus, different groups of people are differentially incorporated into host societies within a hierarchy of citizenship that is shaped by a number of factors, including mode of entry (Stasiulis 2008, 96). The increasing weight that policies in developed countries give to temporary worker programs is of particular importance in the complexity of the migration regime and the privileging of "skilled workers" (101).

Nursing Shortages and the Canadian Welfare State[3]

In Canada, not only is public health care provision a central pillar of the welfare state but it also occupies a critical place within the national imaginary. As the Commission on the Future of Health Care in Canada (Romanow Commission) states: "Canadians embrace medicare as a public good, a national symbol and a defining aspect of their citizenship" (Romanow Commission 2002, xviii).[4] Armstrong and Armstrong (2008, 33) argue that health care is the social program that distinguishes Canadians from Americans. Medicare, they point out, "is a symbol implying we care for each other. It recognizes that we have a shared responsibility as well as a shared risk of ill health. It symbolizes a commitment to health care as a human right, open to all." Consequently, on the one hand, health care is discursively constructed as sacrosanct – a fundamental element of social citizenship; on the other hand, this did not insulate health care in Canada from the neoliberal-inspired reforms of the 1990s, which led to significant restructuring in the public sector. As nurses constitute the largest proportion of workers in the health-care sector (Pyper 2004, 5), they were significantly affected by recent rounds of neoliberal restructuring.

Because of the unique nature of the health sector, states play a critical role in both the supply and the demand of health workers: "Most employment remains in the public sector, but conditions have tended to worsen (relatively and sometimes absolutely) with restructuring" (Connell 2008, 2). During the 1990s, health-care provision in Canada was directly affected by public spending cuts and a concomitant reduction in the provision of social care. The public portion of the total health bill supported by the federal government declined significantly (McBride 2001, 95). While health-care restructuring affects other OECD countries, "The scope of the reduction in public health expenditures appears to be more marked in Canada ... public expenditures as a share of GDP went from a high 7.3% in 1992 to a low 6.2% in 1997, before increasing again and reaching almost 7% in 2005" (Dumont et al. 2008, 16). The Canadian Nurses Association (CNA) reported that there would be a shortfall of 78,000 RNs by 2011 and 113,000 RNs by 2016 (cited by RNAO 2008, 8). Measures introduced in the 1990s contributed significantly to the current shortage of nurses. The dimensions of this shortfall are multifaceted.

Cuts and downsizing in the health sector resulted in job loss. The 1990s witnessed "the largest employment displacement of nurses in recent Canadian history, characterized by massive layoffs as well as sharp increases in casual, part-time, temporary, and contract work" (Grinspun 2003, cited in RNAO 2008, 7). Job losses were, in turn, accompanied by a reorganization of the terms and conditions of work that was inspired by for-profit management techniques. As a result, "nurses [were] made to work harder and faster with fewer others around to help" (Armstrong and Armstrong 2008, 114). Not surprisingly, "two-thirds of RNs reported being very or somewhat stressed in each of the years between 1999 and 2001" (Pyper 2004, 11). In sum, as Kingma (2006, 28) puts it: "Nursing became a lost paradise for those nurses who remained in health care and had to cope with greatly increased workloads, stress, and job dissatisfaction."

The deteriorating conditions of the nursing-care market in Canada play a critical role in the emigration of Canadian nurses to the United States in this same period (see Gabriel 2008): "Overall approximately, 27,000 RNs migrated to the US in the 1990s (Industry Canada, 1999) representing 15 Canadian RNs for every US RN migrating to Canada" (Baumann et al. 2004, 22, citing Zhao, Drew, and Murray 2000). Studies conducted at the time reveal that a key push factor for nurse emigration was a lack of job opportunities, including full-time work (RNAO 2008, 7). The emigration of nurses from Canada to the United States is likely to continue and to exert pressure on the nursing labour force in Canada. Forecasts suggest that the United States will experience a nursing shortage of 800,000 nurses by 2020. For this reason, nurse emigration from Canada to the United States will likely continue (Little 2007, 1339).

Finally, Canada's nursing shortage is linked to changing demographics. The demand for health care and nurses is growing as the baby boom generation ages. At the same time, the nursing labour force is also growing older. The average age of an employed nurse in Canada is 43.7 (Buchan and Calman 2004, 23). To maintain current levels and to accommodate increasing demands for nursing services, the nursing labour force needs to expand and student numbers need to increase substantially in Canada (Kingma 2006, 35). Nevertheless, enrolment in nursing programs "fell from almost 40,000 in 1990-91 to 28,800 in 1998-99" (Pyper 2004, citing Galarneau

2003). This drop reflects provincial cuts to nursing school enrolments starting in 1993, undertaken as part of the broader fiscal restraint package (Little 2007, 1343). More recently, there has been some change on this front and enrolments have risen, with the number of entry-to-practice graduates in Canada exceeding nine thousand for the first time in thirty years (RNAO 2008, 8). This said, nursing shortages are still projected for Canada.

The shortfall of nurses has been in the making for some time. Policy responses to this deficit in care have been framed in terms of improving and retaining the domestic supply of nurses and/or using immigration policy to recruit skilled care workers. Yet, as Little (2007, 1349) notes:

> There appears to be a lack of coherence in the policy approach to addressing the nursing shortage in Canada. Government departments such as labor and immigration are developing policies to address the nursing shortage through immigration while other departments (health) are articulating a solution through increased domestic production, with no substantial coordination between the two.

In line with other nursing organizations, the RNAO supports domestic policy options such as investments in nursing education and improved working conditions. The RNAO and the CNA also advocate supports for IENs who come and work in Canada. In a recent brief, the RNAO (2008, 22) outlines its position: "The individual right to migrate is not in question. What is in question are HHR [health human resources] policies in wealthy countries such as Canada that target HHR from poor countries as a solution to domestically created nursing shortages." Organizations such as the RNAO also raise the issue of the ethics of international recruitment by underscoring the care-related deficits in regions such as Southeast Asia and Africa.

The care deficit in Canada, as this section illustrates, is the outcome of some deliberate policy choices (and policy inaction), not the least of which is a failure to invest in state-organized sectors of reproductive labour, such as nursing. Immigration policy is held up as a means of addressing the nursing shortages, and recent changes within the immigration field, as the next section highlights, do suggest that the federal government is attempting to ease the entry of nurses to Canada. Such efforts should prompt us to think about the parameters of citizenship practice in Canada. To what extent is it acceptable to Canadians that medicare — the sin qua non of social citizenship in Canada — is underpinned by the care work of those who occupy a range of citizenship statuses and may not enjoy the social element of citizenship that T.H. Marshall (1998 [1963], 94) conceptualizes as "the whole range from the right to a modicum of economic welfare and security to the right to share to the full in the social heritage ... according to the standards prevailing in the society." As the shortage of nurses in Canada becomes more critical, the issue of international recruitment will become more salient.

Governing Skilled Care Work: The Case of IENs in Canada

Immigration policy is increasingly touted as a means of addressing skills shortages in key areas of the economy. While control and restrictions remain the hallmark of many immigration regimes in the global economic North (Cornelius et al. 2004), nevertheless, there is an ever-increasing number of admissibility categories that privilege some groups of "desired migrants" (i.e., ideal potential citizens) at the expense of those deemed "less desired." More and more, the differential incorporation of various groups within a hierarchy of citizenship is predicated upon the valorization of the skilled and highly skilled worker. Registered nurses are positioned as skilled workers within this discourse, and the increasing shortage of nurses in Canada would appear to render this occupational category "desired." Recent changes in Canada's immigration regime suggest that the Canadian state and its provincial counterparts are moving to facilitate the entry of nurses by prioritizing them within both permanent and temporary migration streams. Nevertheless, entry to the country as shaped by an immigration regime is only one side of the story. All IENs, whether they enter as permanent migrants or temporary workers, need to complete the requirements for licensure for entry to the profession, and this requirement can pose a significant barrier for some migrant nurses.

The following section considers the ways in which these two aspects of governance — mode of entry to the country and access to a regulated occupation — are implicated in the differential incorporation of IENs into the Canadian health labour market. Consequently, even in the midst of a continuing nursing shortage, many IENs may never work as nurses, finding themselves marginalized from the profession, underemployed or unemployed, while others may be fast tracked to permanent status.

Canadian Institute for Health Information (Canadian Institute for Health Information 2007) data indicate that IENs comprise 7.4 percent of the total RN nursing workforce and that, in Ontario, they account for 11 percent of the total nursing workforce (cited by Kolawole 2009, 185). It is difficult, however, to estimate accurately the actual numbers of registered nurses in Canada with overseas training because Citizenship and Immigration Canada collects data only by applicant category. As a result, it is unclear how many IENs live in Canada. IENs become identified only if they register with a provincial regulatory body (Baumann et al. 2006, 10). "Regulatory bodies reported the following countries in descending order as the most frequent source of IEN applicants: the Philippines, United States, United Kingdom, and Australia" (Little 2007, 1340).

Entry to the Country: The Immigration Regime
In the postwar period, Canadian immigration policy has undergone a series of shifts. In the 1960s, explicit racial preferences were discarded in favour of the more technocratic and rational points-based selection model. By the 1990s, growing emphasis was placed on skilled workers. The "high-skilled" migrant worker came to be represented as the most desirable, unproblematic category of migrant for many countries. Neoliberal assumptions position the skilled migrant worker as a means of enhancing national competitiveness in a globalizing economy (Abu-Laban and Gabriel 2002). Throughout changes in immigration policy, a constant perception is that the country "selects future citizens, not just workers" (Alboim and Maytree 2009, 50), reflecting the role that, historically, immigration has played in nation building (Reitz 2004). Recent initiatives adopted by the Conservative government suggest an increasing emphasis on temporary worker programs. How do recent developments in the immigration regime and preferences for skilled workers frame the entry and status of migrant nurses to Canada? Here, the rules governing the varying modes of entry mean that IENs can have very different experiences of the rights that citizenship entails.

IENs can apply to enter Canada through a variety of permanent and temporary programs. Some provinces and employers do engage in targeted recruitment campaigns; however, most nurses enter Canada as landed immigrants without pre-arranged job offers (Blythe and Baumann 2009, 192). IENs can migrate through the skilled worker category, through provincial nominees programs, through the Canadian Experience Class, through temporary worker programs, or as live-in caregivers. IENs may also enter as refugees or family members. The next section maps some of the modes of entry associated with the immigration regime that regulates nurse migration to Canada.

Permanent Immigration: Federal Skilled Worker Category

The selection of economic migrants has always been linked to labour market imperatives. In the 1960s, Canada pioneered a points-based model to select independent applicants — what are now referred to as skilled workers — within the economic component of the immigration program. Originally, points were awarded in nine categories, including education, age, employment opportunities in Canada, official language ability, and suitability, with the heaviest weighting accorded to occupation and skill categories. The introduction of a points-based model was a break with the explicit discrimination that had characterized previous Canadian policy. As argued elsewhere, however, the selection model still embodies a number of gender, racialized, and class exclusions (Abu-Laban and Gabriel 2002). IENs' experience with this selection model has been mixed, and what comes to the fore is that the points system has not always recognized nursing as a priority occupation.

During the 1990s, the issue of critical skills shortage dominated the public agenda, and immigration was identified as a way to address the need for skilled workers in critical sectors of the economy (Little 2006, 1344). As Stasiulis and Bakan (2003, 110) argue, however, despite apparent nursing shortages, Citizenship and Immigration Canada (CIC) "denied such a shortage existed by awarding zero points to nurses in the General Occupations List (GOL) that determined eligibility for permanent or landed immigrant status. This made it virtually impossible for foreign nurses to acquire sufficient points in order to enter as independent, landed immigrants." The exclusion of nursing occupations from the GOL may have prompted families to designate a principal applicant who was not involved with health care and "who was therefore more likely to be selected." As a result, since 1986, 23 percent of people indicating they wanted to work as registered nurses were dependents (Dumont et al. 2008, 41). It was only in 1997, when the Canadian Nurses Association published a study outlining a projected shortage of RNs by 2011, that the state acknowledged a nursing crisis (Little 2007, 1344).

In an effort to update the immigration system, in 2002 the federal government introduced new legislation: the Immigration Reform and Protection Act (IRPA). While the points-based model was retained, more emphasis was placed on official language ability, education, and work experience, and the GOL was discarded. For this reason, there was some optimism that RNs wishing to apply within the economic class would be more successful. In 2008, the Conservative government announced that it would process the applications of those individuals under the points system only if they:

- Have an offer of arranged employment, or
- [Are] a foreign national living legally in Canada for one year as a temporary foreign worker or an international student, or
- [Are] a skilled worker who has at least one year of experience in one or more of the following occupations. (Citizenship and Immigration Canada 2009)

Registered nurses and other health-related occupations figure among thirty-eight professions listed (Citizenship and Immigration Canada 2009). On the one hand, the addition of RNs to the list is indicative of the critical need for skilled care workers. On the other hand, such recognition is no predictor of getting a job in Canada commensurate with training and experience.

The current application process has been criticized for obscuring the difficulties in the attendant credentialing process (Alboim and Maytree 2009, 33). The evaluation of education, training, and skills within the points system leaves accepted applicants with the impression that they will be able to enter the Canadian labour market with some degree of ease because their knowledge and credentials will be recognized (Jeans et al. 2005, 24). Yet, nursing is one of the top twenty regulated professions in Canada, and the demands associated with licensure often prove to be a formidable barrier. Some nurses have reported that they were provided with insufficient information about how to re-establish their careers (Baumann et al. 2006, 15). Others reported that they were given poor information. For example:

> The guy there that interviewed us told my husband, "You're going to have a hard time finding a job. But, you, on the other hand, you're a nurse. It's easy for you to get a job there." And my husband is like, "Oh great. We'll go." But then when I came here, I was shocked. You know there's a nursing shortage here, but they won't easily hire you if you don't have the right connections, stuff like this (IEN). (Baumann et al. 2006, 15)

Permanent Immigration: Provincial Nominee Programs

Among the most significant changes in Canada's immigration architecture is the growth of provincial nominee programs (PNPs). Since 1998, all provinces have signed federal/provincial/territorial accords or PNPs related to the management of migration. These agreements allow provinces to bypass the national points-based model and fast-track those applicants constructed as critical for the functioning of local and provincial economies. Provincial nominees are given priority in these processes, and there is no limit to the numbers provinces may select. These admissions have grown rapidly from "less than 500 to over 22,000 over an eight year period" (Alboim and Maytree 2009, 16). It has been suggested that, while these programs were designed to "complement the Federal Skilled Worker Program," they are now well on the "way to replacing it" (35). All PNPs are employer-driven, and four jurisdictions (i.e., British Columbia, Newfoundland, Ontario, and Saskatchewan) have either specific categories or programs that target the health-care sector. CIC has also developed a pilot project with the Province of Alberta that uses the PNP to fast-track the applications of doctors, nurses, physiotherapists, and pharmacists whose applications are pending in the federal skilled-worker category (Dumont et al. 2008, 43).

Recent changes in the federal skilled worker program and the growth of PNPs, many of which target health workers, facilitate the entry of nurses and are indicative of the increasing importance of skilled care workers to Canada. In the period from 2002 to 2006, the permanent migration of nurses increased by 39 percent (Dumont et al. 2008, 42). Canadian permanent resident status provides IENS access to social rights, such as employment standards protection, human rights legislation, and so on, and, if they have the means, eligibility to sponsor family members. Permanent residents enjoy all the rights guaranteed by the Canadian Charter of Rights and Freedoms, and, after a period of time, permanent residents can apply for Canadian citizenship.

Temporary Migration

Canada's immigration architecture also includes the Temporary Foreign Worker Program (TFWP), which includes programs that target both low- and high-skilled workers as well as sector-specific programs. The Seasonal Agricultural Workers Program and the Live-in-Caregiver Program are examples of sector-specific programs that have a long history in Canada. Under the rules of these programs, workers are generally permitted to enter Canada for a fixed period of time on the proviso that employers demonstrate they have made an effort to hire Canadians according to prevailing market conditions, which is verified through a labour market opinion conducted by Human Resources and Skills Development Canada (HRSDC) (Service Canada) (Alboim and Maytree 2009, 36). Since coming to power, the Conservative government has moved to promote and expand this program. In the period from 2004 to 2008, initial entries of temporary workers have gone up by 71.2 percent, and, in 2008, some provinces (i.e., British Columbia, Alberta, Newfoundland and Labrador, and the Territories) received more temporary workers than permanent residents (18). The employment of temporary workers can be characterized as precarious because it is largely predicated on their status as non-citizens. Workers in this category are required to return to countries of origin, may have difficulties availing themselves of rights and status, and suffer from a lack of oversight regarding employer practices. Additionally, the status of temporary workers renders them ineligible for state-funded immigrant settlement and language programs (27-28).

IENs do enter Canada under the auspices of the TFWP. In contrast to the prevailing trends, however, the number of RN temporary entries has always been smaller than that of permanent entries. During most of the 1990s, there were zero temporary recruitments (Dumont et al. 2008, 40). In 2006, 240 nurses entered the country as temporary foreign workers. Between 2002 and 2006, the number of temporary entries decreased by 34 percent (42). As noted above, nurses who come to Canada on a temporary basis must have their offers of employment confirmed by the HRSDC through the instrument of a labour market opinion (Baumann et al. 2004, 11). Since 2006, however, the HRSDC has generated "Regional Occupations Under Pressure lists" to recognize occupations "that are facing labour market pressure" (Dumont et al. 2008, 43). In the case of identified occupations, employers do not have to engage in a labour market search before applying to hire a temporary worker. Such lists are now in operation in Alberta, British Columbia, Manitoba, Nova Scotia, Ontario, Prince Edward Island, and Quebec. All but two provinces have included RNs on the list (Dumont et al. 2008, 43). In the context of growing recourse to temporary work permits and looming shortages in the health sector, this aspect of immigration policy warrants further investigation.

Canadian Experience Class

The Canadian government recently announced a new route to permanent resident status: the Canadian Experience Class (CEC). Under its terms, foreign student graduates and some temporary workers in Canada become eligible to apply for permanent residence on the proviso that they have twenty-four months of work experience. This new category prioritizes skill in so far as eligibility is largely determined by "professional, managerial and skilled work experience." Prospective applicants would also need to demonstrate some language skills (Citizenship and Immigration Canada 2008b). The new program offers a route to permanent resident status for some temporary workers and foreign students, but it effectively bars temporary foreign workers in what are considered low-skilled or unskilled jobs from taking advantage of this option. The CEC was implemented in the fall of 2008. Initial take-up was slow (Keung 2008), but, according to CIC's Annual Report to Parliament, the government planned to admit between five thousand and seventy-five hundred applicants in 2009 (Citizenship and Immigration Canada 2008a).

It has been suggested that, with its emphasis on skilled occupations, the CEC will have a differential impact on men and women. According to CIC 2006 statistics, 51.1 percent of men working on temporary work permits would qualify for this program, while only 22 percent of women with temporary work permits would be eligible (CCR 2008, 3). IENs will be in this group because registered nursing falls into a skilled occupation that requires a university education. Further, IENs in this category have met the existing credentialing requirements necessary for working in Canada, leading one report to surmise: "the selection of what amounts to 'pre-integrated' persons will yield better labour market outcomes for immigrants in general" (Dumont et al. 2008, 44). This said, some non-governmental groups, drawing on the case of live-in caregivers, caution: "The two years of work required before being able to apply under the CEC makes workers more vulnerable to employer abuse, as they may be reluctant to report abuse so as not to jeopardize their chances of obtaining permanent status"(CCR 2008, 3). In effect, the CEC provides a path towards "earned citizenship." While IENs, in contrast to many low-skilled, temporary workers, will be able to avail themselves of this opportunity, the condition of full-time employment and their temporary status places them in a precarious position.

The Live-In Caregiver Program

Canada's Live-In Caregiver Program (LCP) provides the clearest example of how barriers imposed by immigration policy, the workings of a temporary work program, and credentialing all come together to create a situation in which skilled migrant women caregivers experience downward occupational mobility, a loss of skills, and partial citizenship.

The LCP occupies a unique position within Canada's immigration architecture because it is a program designed explicitly to permit Canadian families to recruit non-Canadian female domestic workers to provide care work in the private realm of the home. Under the terms of the LCP — implemented in 1992 and currently under review — migrant women workers must have completed the equivalent of high school and be able to speak

English or French. They are required to live in the homes of their employers. It is the latter aspect more than any other that renders workers vulnerable to long hours and employer abuse. While domestic workers are formally covered by employment standards legislation regarding wages, hours, and overtime, there are problems regarding monitoring, compliance, and enforcement of contracts (Langevin and Belleau 2000). In the period from 1993 to 2006, 35,719 women and 919 men entered Canada under the LCP. Most female caregivers were between the ages of twenty-five and forty-four. A majority of these workers (83 percent) held Philippine citizenship (Spitzer and Torres 2008, 10-13).

The LCP is "distinguished" from other programs because it holds out the promise of permanent resident status (and, ultimately, Canadian citizenship) on the condition that foreign domestic workers complete twenty-four months of employment in a three-year period from the time they land in Canada. This aspect of the program is directly related to migrant workers' ability to claim rights. Workers and their employers are aware that the former "are 'on probation' for at least two years. This creates a disincentive for live-in caregivers to insist on their employment rights" (Macklin 2002, 231). This is because to do so might jeopardize one's current and future citizenship status. Yet, as Spitzer and Torres (2008, 14) show, contract violations – for example, "non-payment of salary, unpaid and unlimited overtime; the inability to take sick leave; substandard housing arrangements ... being compelled to do tasks prohibited by the contract including farm work" – are well documented.

The points-based immigration model did not recognize nursing as one of its listed professions on the GOL in the 1990s, and, as a result, IENs could not enter Canada under the independent class provision. It is suggested that this is the reason that many nurses trained in the Philippines entered Canada under the terms of the LCP (Langevin and Belleau 2000, 37). Many of these women experienced subsequent de-skilling and downward mobility.

As Spitzer and Torres (2008, 14) state: "Invariably, LCP workers come to Canada with the intention of recovering their careers or continuing their education after they have completed the Program; however, policies that constrain opportunities for retraining while under the Program, and financial pressures stemming from the need to place familial priorities ahead of their own, often mean that they must put their own dreams on hold." Registered nursing offers a case in point. It has been noted that the terms and conditions of domestic work affect the ability of IENs to take courses or adequately prepare for the licensing exam. Further, they cannot apply to take the exam until they secure permanent residence status, by which time they will not have practised nursing for some time (Baumann et al. 2006, 15). IENs who enter through the LCP are often unable to meet a critical requirement for licensure, namely, that they must have "have practiced for a minimum of time in the previous 3-5 years to maintain currency [requirement ranges from 800 to 1,685 hours of needed experience]" (Dumont et al. 2008, 59). As a result, they may delay or abandon nursing altogether (Baumann et al. 2006, 15). Filipino women's groups, such as the Filipino Nurses Support Group, have tried to raise awareness that the LCP results in downward mobility.

Entry to a Regulated Profession
The experience of IENs in Canada is not only shaped and regulated by the modes of entry associated with the national immigration architecture but is also determined by the ability (or lack of ability) to gain entry to the profession of registered nursing. Thus, the movement of migrant nurses in a global care market is also framed by the workings of regulatory bodies and institutions in destination countries that verify credentials and skills obtained by nurses in sending countries. Currently, there "is no internationally recognized and accepted standard that governs nurse licensure"; each country and/or state and province determines what training and skills are required (Kingma 2006, 95). Consequently, as Yeates (2009, 110) notes, "the need for certification can impede access to national health labour markets."

The processes entailed in securing registration in Canada have proven to be a barrier to entry to the profession (Kolawole 2009). The regulation of registered nurses in Canada is conducted at the level of provinces and territories, which, in, turn delegate responsibility to a professional body. In Ontario, for example, a number of steps must be completed in the application process for licensure:

- Completion of an acceptable RN ... educational programme,
- Recent safe nursing practice,
- Passing the RN ... examination,
- Language fluency,
- Registration or eligibility for registration in the jurisdiction of the completed nursing programme,
- Canadian citizenship or permanent resident status, as well as
- Good character and Canadian criminal record synopsis. (Kolawole 2009, 185).

The College of Nurses of Ontario is responsible for verifying credentials (i.e., application form and submission of documents) through an examination of documents. Relevant documents for all RN regulatory bodies include: "completed application forms, proof of language proficiency, verification of original registration in home country, verification of current registration. Nine out of 10 require marriage/birth certificates, course transcripts, passport or photo identification" (Jeans et al. 2005, 26). This process of securing relevant documents can be lengthy: applicants experience difficulties obtaining documents from home countries, and incomplete paperwork was cited by regulators as one of the key reasons for failed applications (26-28). Moreover, many IENs may not be aware of the requirements of licensure and, as a result, fail to bring all documents with them when migrating (Kolawole 2009, 185). Finally, IENs would have to assume costs of the application process, which may include: "translation, examination fees, language tests and the cost of tuition for refresher courses and/or bridging programs," all of which would be significant for those who are unemployed or underemployed (Jeans et al. 2005, 40).

In the period from 1999 to 2003, only 50 percent of IENs (RNs) were eligible to write the exam (Jeans et al. 2005, 33). An applicant is eligible to write the licensing examination after her documents are accepted and her education is recognized as equivalent to that of a Canadian graduate. Once eligibility is determined, IENS need to write a licensing exam designed to "measure the competencies that Canadian nurses have identified as necessary for safe and effective nursing practice," yet many of them have not been successful on their initial attempt (Baumann et al. 2006, 21-22). High failure rates have been linked to cultural and language barriers (Jeans et al. 2005, 40).

Not passing the exam means that IENs will not be able to practise their profession in Ontario. Regulatory bodies seek to ensure that the nursing competencies of IENs are equivalent to those of a Canadian-trained nurse. Consequently, as Jeans et al. argue, such bodies perceive their role as safeguarding and protecting the public interest. Most regulatory bodies do not consider facilitating the entry of IENS to the profession through the use of education/bridging programs as part of their mandate, but this, too, could be seen as being in the public interest (Jeans et al. 2005, 44).

The regulatory framework governing entry to the profession limits the ability of IENs to gain access to the nursing profession: the individual skills of a migrant care worker must be formally recognized in the form of professional accreditation. Some RNs will not be able to work as RNs in Canada because they were unable or unwilling to write a qualifying exam, while others will be unable to pass the exam. The non-recognition of qualifications and training earned abroad results in a process of de-skilling as IENs may find themselves either underemployed or unemployed. As Boyd and Pikkov (2008, 41) point out, although IENs may earn more in Canada and the United States than in their home countries, they may also be in more vulnerable positions, be employed as nurses' aides rather than RNs, and may "experience discrimination on the job in the form of lower pay, fewer promotions and may be readily fired." Further, while entry to the labour market is important for financial well-being, it is also "critical to integration, identity formation, ability to claim a sense of belonging and ultimately, full citizenship" (Galabuzi 2005, 53).

Conclusion

This chapter uses the case of IENs in Canada to highlight the role a nation-state plays in shaping women's transnational care migration. The entry of IENs to the country is governed by an increasingly stratified migration regime that draws sharp distinctions between categories of admissibility and, by extension, the rights associated with formal citizenship. Consequently, IENs can occupy contradictory or hierarchal citizenship positions predicated on their mode of entry. IENs who enter under the terms of the skilled-worker category have entrée to a range of economic, social, and political entitlements, while those who are admitted as live-in caregivers have limited employment mobility and residence rights. The mode of entry also may affect the ability of IENs to enter the labour market.

New directions within immigration categories have prioritized RNs on occupations lists at the federal and provincial levels, reflecting the increasing demand for skilled caregivers. Yet the prominence of temporary work programs and "earned" avenues to permanent migration, such as the Canadian Experience Class, also render skilled migrant care workers vulnerable to workplace exploitation. Further, entry to the country, whether as permanent residents or as temporary workers, is a separate process from licensure, which governs entry to the regulated profession of nursing. Consequently, while registered nurses are regarded as skilled workers (and, indeed, desired workers), for the purposes of entry to the country, there is no guarantee that the procedures associated with the nursing licensure process will permit entry to the profession. Indeed, in the Canadian case, there seems to be a disjuncture between recent directions in immigration policy, which appear to create opportunities for nurse migration, and the measures regulating access to the profession. As a result, one outcome of this disjuncture is the marginalization of many IENs within the nursing profession.

The "crisis of care" that many countries in the global North are experiencing is deeply implicated in the ongoing restructuring of care labour on a global scale. The transnational movement of care workers, such as nurses, is an integral part of this restructuring and is shaped not only by processes of globalization but also by the national citizenship and immigration policies and practices of individual states.

3

The Global Migration of Care Labour
Filipino Workers in Japan

HIRONORI ONUKI

This chapter focuses on the implications of a new agreement between Japan and the Philippines as a way of exploring the contradictions and tensions surrounding the migration of Filipino care workers to Japan, where, as Yuki Tsuji (this volume) argues, a rapid expansion of the aging population accompanied by a dramatic shrinkage of the Japanese labour force has triggered heated debates over how to cope with the acute demand for elder "care."[1] The Japan-Philippines Economic Partnership Agreement (JPEPA) – the bilateral Economic Partnership Agreement [EPA] signed in September 2006 and ratified in December 2008, which allows for the Philippines to send up to four hundred nurses and six hundred care workers to Japan over a period of two years (MOFA 2006) – was described in the Japanese media as "[a] new step toward opening Japan's labour market" (*Asahi Shimbun* 2006). The government of Japan has also signed a similar EPA with Indonesia, which includes the same clause, permitting Indonesian nurses and care workers to work in Japan (MOFA 2007b).[2] Given Japan's strict immigration regulations regarding the entry of so-called "unskilled" workers,[3] such deregulation of the inflows of "foreign" labour to Japan is remarkable, especially in terms of care workers whose professional status has not yet been verified in the Japanese labour market (Son 2007; Takagi 2006).

These developments need to be placed within the wider context of how the neoliberal transformations in capitalist relations of production and social reproduction have not only reorganized gender order (Bakker 1999;

Pearson 2004; Peterson 2003) but have also created the "globalization of care work" – that is, the gendered, racialized, and classed "international division of reproductive labour" – through the migration of mainly female workers from the global South to the global North (Misra et al. 2006; Parreñas 2001a, 2005a). Built upon these ontological and epistemological conceptions, this chapter addresses the following questions: First, how far and in what ways has the neoliberal shift towards more market-oriented governance of the global political economy involved the commodification and transnationalization of relations of social reproduction? Second, how far and in what ways does the international division of reproductive labour promote and/or constrain the (re)formation of identity and political subjectivity among transnational migrant care workers? I argue that the "deployment" of Filipino care workers in Japan contributes to a hierarchical regime of social reproduction based on gender, nationality, class, ethnicity, and/or "race."

The first section of this chapter maps the content of the JPEPA, placing special emphasis on how Japan's official view of the reception of Filipino workers as its "special present" to the Philippines shapes the subject formation of Filipino care migrants. The next section, while utilizing the various narratives of actual and potential Filipino migrant care workers, brings attention to the prospective contestations and/or negotiations of these labourers within the emerging social spaces for their everyday lives of working and living in Japan.[4]

The JPEPA and Japan's "Special Present"

> *The decision to accept Filipino care workers and nurses into Japan is the special present from the Japanese government to its Philippine counterpart.*
>
> – *Official, Japan's Ministry of Health, Labour and Welfare*[5]

According to the JPEPA, the program's main objective is to contribute to the shared development of medical and social welfare in both countries (MHLW 2006). Since the JPEPA does not allow for mutual recognition of national licences, Filipino care workers are candidates to become *kaigo fukushishi* (certified care workers) in Japan.[6] They must have graduated with a four-year university degree and, in addition, in most cases, have received a caregiver's certificate issued by the Technical Education and Skills Development

Authority (TESDA) of the Philippine government. The candidates selected by the Philippine government agencies have to enrol in a six-month program in Japan, consisting of language education and caregiving preparation and given at the Association for Overseas Technical Scholarship (AOTS)/ Japan Foundation. The training costs are covered by Japan's official development assistance (ODA) fund. After this, they undergo on-the-job training (OJT) for a maximum of four years, signing employment contracts with the care institutions approved by the Japan International Corporation of Welfare Services (JICWEL), a semi-governmental organization sanctioned by the Ministry of Health, Labour, and Welfare (MHLW). Their remuneration is to be commensurable with that of their Japanese counterparts performing the same tasks. Upon completing the three-year OJT, they will take Japan's national licence examination in Japanese. After passing the examination, Filipino candidates will be able to work in Japan as *kaigo fukushishi* for another three years (which will be renewable), but those who fail must leave Japan by the end of their four-year visa terms.

State ministries have held conflicting views concerning the "movements of people," especially of care workers, in the EPAs. The Japanese Ministry of Economy, Trade, and Industry proposes the creation of a mutual recognition system for the qualification of care workers as it regards the successful establishment of the EPAs with its neighbours as vital to sustaining Japan's global competitiveness (METI 2006). The Nihon Keidanren (Japan Business Federation), composed of Japan's leading companies, similarly favours the expansion of the EPAs and the active acceptance of "foreign" care workers to manage a sharply rising demand for care labour (Wajima 2005). In contrast, denying the existence of a labour shortage in Japan's caregiving sector, the MHLW (2005a) claims that the inflow of "foreign" care labour to Japan must be limited in order to prevent any negative impact on the Japanese labour market. As this stance dominated during the negotiation of the JPEPA, the introduction of Filipino care workers has been considered as Japan's "exceptional" political compromise in accommodating the overall parameters of the EPA – its "special present" to the Philippines.

From this viewpoint, whereas the reception of Filipino care workers in Japan is seen as a minor exception, as reflected in the limited quota of six hundred candidates over two years, its primary objective is to "secure care work forces domestically" by mobilizing the potential workers who hold certificates but who are not currently engaged in caregiving jobs and by improving working conditions in this sector.[7] Nevertheless, the alarmingly high share of the elderly (one in every five Japanese was sixty-five and older in 2007) along with a very low birth rate (1.32 in 2006) has sharply escalated the need for care labour (Cabinet Office 2008b; MHLW 2007a).[8] Nobue Suzuki (2007, 361-62) posits that the MHLW's denial of the necessity of "foreign" care workers is based on the idea that caring for the elderly is a familial obligation, underpinned by the "institutional gender division of labour" — women as primary care providers in families, working out of "love" — which has played an instrumental role in Japan's postwar economic growth. While this belief is still reflected in Japan's recent policy reforms for the reprivatization of care work, since the late 1980s, the state has begun to recognize the rise of the nuclear family and the growing feminization of labour. The Japanese state has paradoxically expedited a readjustment from family-based to socially shared care provision for the elderly by constructing what Kiyoe Sugimoto (1998) terms the "new Japanese-style welfare society." This discourse of the "socialization of care," as Tsuji (this volume) suggests, makes the practices of caregiving socially visible as paid labour and serves as a motivating force behind their marketization, formalized with the long-term care insurance (LTCI) system begun in 2000.

With the launch of LTCI, which involves the deregulation of the welfare sector and encourages the entry of private companies into the marketized care services, the accelerated commodification of care labour has resulted in the deterioration of working conditions in the caregiving sector, which has been socially devalued as feminized reproductive jobs associated with the image of "3K" (*kitanai, kitsui,* and *kyuryo/kyuka sukunai* — dirty, difficult, and low salary/vacation) (Sawami 2005). The marketization of care work has induced the utilization of "flexible" low-wage part-time and contract workers (mainly female and young) to reduce labour costs, thus augmenting unstable, insecure employment. These trends, together with the physical and mental requirements of supplying "high-quality" care services in market competitions, have resulted in high turnover rates among care workers (20.2 percent in 2006, which is high in comparison to other sectors) (Inoue 2005; Sawami 2006). Managers and workers at care institutions have complained about understaffing (*Asahi Shimbun* 2008).

Given the striking gap between the state's claim of "securing care labour domestically" and the impending severe labour shortages in (re)privatized and marketized care work, the scheme outlined in the JPEPA appears to establish a solid basis for the introduction of Filipino care labour by setting various conditions for the recipient institutions, including certain numbers of certified care workers and the capacity to provide sufficient training and assistance. As some people at care facilities note, however, only a very limited number of well-staffed institutions can afford to meet such provisions (Sawami 2007, 161). Indeed, although the JICWEL is assigned to cope with the welfare of Filipino candidates, the details of its services (e.g., the arrangement of Tagalog-speaking counsellors) have yet to be decided (Suzuki 2007, 367). Of crucial importance is the stipulation that Filipino candidates must acquire Japan's *kaigo fukushishi* certificate in order to work after their initial four-year term. While it is doubtful whether the intensive six-month language training at AOTS will sufficiently equip Filipinos to "work" in Japanese-speaking caregiving environments,[9] what is even more problematic is whether these workers will be able to pass the written exam in Japanese: in 2006, the pass rate was only 47 percent even among Japanese nationals (MHLW 2007b). In other words, although the introduction of Filipino care labour to Japan under the JPEPA could be regarded as increasing migration and settlement (Asato 2007, 38), it creates high barriers, potentially preventing a large number of Filipinos from settling in Japan. Thus, Japan's official conception of the reception of Filipino care-worker candidates to Japan as a "special present" to the Philippines not only fails to ameliorate immanent care labour needs but also compels Filipinos (especially those without Japanese licences) to become "cheap" labour sources. If the inflows of Filipino care labour to Japan are expanded with the (re)privatization of elder care provision, the JPEPA can arguably be seen to systematize the short-term supply of racialized "flexible" and "disposable" reproductive workers to fill Japan's impending vacuum of "gendered" and socially "unfavourable" labour.

The next section directs attention towards how Filipino migrant care workers have experienced and will experience the implications of these neoliberal arrangements in their everyday lives. It attempts to expose the prospective struggles, contestations, and negotiations of these workers, drawing on Louise Amoore's conceptualization of globalization as contested social practices as well as on insights provided by the work of Henri Lefebvre and Rhacel Salazar Parreñas.

The Everyday Spaces of Filipino Care Workers with "Partial Citizenship" in Japan

Amoore (2002) elucidates the ways in which the emerging social relations of neoliberal globalization constitute, and are shaped by, the structured social practices that make these changes possible. It is the everyday practices of workers that make particular forms of global production possible and that potentially shape contested and contradictory dynamics of social change in current and future conditions. Thus, the structural transformations of the global political economy need to be seen as contested and as contingent upon the structured everyday practices of individuals and groups at multiple levels. From this practice-centred perspective of global politics, it is possible to view Filipino care workers not as passive but as active subjects. To further illuminate the multilayered and multifaceted practices of the transnational transfer of Filipino care labour to Japan, Lefebvre's concepts of "everyday life" and "social space" are useful.

For Lefebvre (1991 [1974], 73; see also Lefebvre 1991 [1947]), "everyday life" is a contested place characterized by mystifications that derive from the experience of alienation in modern society and the struggle to overcome them, while "space" is socially produced as the precondition and the outcome of practices "that permit fresh action to occur, while suggesting others and prohibiting yet others." Given these conceptualizations, Lefebvre sees the possibility of emancipatory action in recognizing the contradictions between the actual experience of everyday life and the ideological claims made about it – the contradictions that are mystified through the process of extending abstract space (in his view, the space of capitalism) into all spheres of human life. Working from Lefebvre's insistence that lived spaces are strategic locations in which the social struggle may overcome such mystifications, Matt Davies and Michael Niemann (2002, 567) stress that "we must account for the waxing and waning of the capacities of specific social agents to effect global politics, and for the circulation of struggles among different actors and between the various levels of social life." Following Lefebvre, they argue that everyday life occurs in the concrete lived spaces people make for themselves and that it is composed of a dialectical unity/totality involving family, work, and leisure. These three social spaces are viewed as crucial arenas in which one's emancipatory potential can be pursued. Here, it is important not to romanticize Filipino care workers as unobstructed political subjects but, rather, to concretize their everyday struggles with the structures shaping their introduction to Japan, especially as they are shaped by what Parreñas calls "partial citizenship."

In reflecting on the paradoxical situations of transnational Filipino migrant domestic workers in various industrialized societies around the globe, Parreñas (2001b) shows how the "contradictory regulatory practices" of receiving nation-states impose the subject positioning of partial citizenship on these workers. Built upon T.H. Marshall's conception of citizenship, the notion of "partial citizenship" describes the limited incorporation of low-wage labour migrants — both male and female — into their receiving societies. Migrant Filipina domestic workers "provide care for the citizenry of various receiving nations at the cost of the denial of their own reproduction (most receiving nations deny citizenship to the children of migrant Filipina domestics) and membership in the nation-state that they are reproducing" (Parreñas 2001b, 1130). Hence, it is crucial to analyze the social practices of introducing Filipino care workers to Japan, and these workers' prospective everyday contestations and negotiations within the social spaces of family, work, and leisure, by asking the question: how far and in what ways do their experiences as transnational care workers in Japanese society embody the idea of partial citizenship – that is, of discriminately stunted social, economic, and political rights?

The Social Spaces of Family, Motivations, and Social Rights

Many Filipino care workers and students at the caregiver training schools take caregiving courses with the aim of seeking overseas employment. Johnny,[10] a male caregiving student with a bachelor of arts in engineering and communication, describes his situation: "Since I graduated with a non-medical degree, I could not imagine myself doing caregiving job before. But, these days, we all know the economic situation of the Philippines, and that being employed here is not well compensated. That is why we look for possible ways to work abroad, not professional, such as doctor or engineer. So, caregiver! That is why so many of us are taking up caregiving." For most who become transnational migrant labour, working as caregivers abroad is regarded as the easiest way to overcome the limited financial options available to them in the Philippines. Filipinos' motivations to acquire overseas job opportunities frequently stem from the importance of obligatory and reciprocal familial relations in the Philippines. In particular, "for a woman to be mindful of the well-being of her family, primarily parents but also dependent siblings, fulfils one of the dictates of Philippine femininity" (Barber 2000, 402). Glenda, a single female certified caregiver training at Tropical Paradise Village (TPV) in Subic Bay, Philippines – a residential treatment facility for retired Japanese, where Filipino caregivers prepare for working in Japan – explains why she intends to work abroad as a caregiver: "This is for my family, particularly for my parents. When they become elderly, I want to provide them with something that they could not obtain during their young age. I want to help them financially and provide a comfortable life for them." Thus, it would appear that providing "help" to parents and relatives through remittances may influence labour migration decision making among Filipinas.

Indeed, many Filipina mothers see transnational labour migration as the most viable means of ensuring that their children receive a solid education (e.g., *Shimotsuke Shimbun* 2007a). This is exemplified by the narrative of Maria, a caregiving student who, as a single mother, raised a twelve-year-old son upon returning to the Philippines after four and a half years in Japan and divorcing her Japanese husband. In her words: "I think that while working abroad I may be able to save some money for the future ... I want to give my kid the best education, because I believe that that is the only way to provide him a good future. This is impossible to do ... while I am working in the Philippines. So, we are very eager to work abroad." As these narratives show, the emergence of women — both daughters and mothers — whose remittances situate them as family breadwinners has posed challenges to the historically constructed sexual division of labour in Philippine society (Eviota 1992, 145). These stories not only highlight how financial insecurity results in Filipino households' sending able-bodied members abroad as transnational care workers but also indicate a degree of agency on the part of migrant workers themselves. Given this, TPV president Nobuyuki Takahashi criticizes the main JPEPA debates for focusing exclusively on whether Japan should accept the flow of Filipino care workers. This ignores the possible problems these workers may encounter while working abroad. One of the questions that needs to be addressed concerns "how to deal with the family issue while Filipinos are working in Japan and separating from their own families."[11]

This silence in the JPEPA follows from the Japanese state's perception of Filipino care workers as an "exceptional case." From the employers' viewpoint, "foreign" migrant labourers with temporary residence permits may be preferred largely because, being separated from their families, they are able to conduct their jobs without distraction. However, while these migrant care workers help to reproduce social relations of (re)production within the neoliberalized Japanese political economy, their own social reproductive rights are likely to be restricted. The practice of family separation generates the phenomenon of transnational households, posing the question of who is to care for those left behind in the Philippines. In other words, under the JPEPA, the perception of Filipino care workers as temporary residents and the implicit limits placed on family reunification leads not only to placing the responsibility for reproducing care labourers outside of Japan but also to making Filipino migrants racially differentiated and discriminated subjects, whose reproduction is not allowed in Japanese society, despite their contributions to its reproduction.

Under the JPEPA, the restriction on the social reproductive rights of Filipino care workers generates few incentives for Filipinos to work in Japan when some nation-states, including Canada and the United States, offer them family reunification policies. Consider the case of Genalyn, a student enrolled in the Canadian live-in caregiver program in Manila, whose husband has worked as a waiter on international cruise ships for the last eleven years: "[Japan] is not attractive for me. Honestly speaking, I have no intention of going to Japan. My main reason for working abroad is to bring my family there. After working in Japan for two years and needing to come back here, we will have nothing to start on. In this context, my husband still needs to work abroad, while being apart from our family." Should Filipino care workers such as Genalyn decide to come to Japan, they may see the latter as a stepping stone to another nation, one whose state regulations and social conditions offer better opportunities for family reunification (Suzuki 2007, 373). This possibility raises the question of whether Filipinos, who are largely English-speaking and currently employed in various nations across the world, would be willing to come to work in Japan when doing so would entail their learning the Japanese language. Nevertheless, Carmina B-Dimayuga, a member of the staff of the VGB Center for Training and Development Corporation (a caregiving school in Quezon City, Philippines), indicates how Japan is considered an attractive option for Filipino students. According to her, when this school provided the Japan-focused "Healthcare Provider Course" in 2005-06, it had 250 Filipino graduates. She says that the school has been receiving a large number of inquiries from prospective students who are looking for working in Japan.[12]

When looking at Filipinos' motivation to become transnational care workers, it is important to consider the ways in which Filipino caregivers/caregiving trainees have internalized the discourse of "caring Filipinos," which is widely mobilized by the Philippine state (Ito et al. 2005). In explaining their choice of caregiving as an occupation, many designate caring as an innate trait of Filipinos. Interestingly, so do Japanese business groups. Concerning this "coincidence," Suzuki (2007, 376) notes: "Filipino careworkers' 'innate abilities' and adaptability to the emerging social conditions may be conveniently cast into the changing structure of work and caregiving in Japan." This idea may be further developed by examining the social spaces of work for Filipino care labourers coming to Japan, along with their economic rights.

The Social Spaces of Work, Classed/Racial Stratification, and Economic Rights

Some Filipino care workers worked in Japan, within the so-called grey zone, before the introduction of the JPEPA.[13] Allan, a certified Filipino caregiver, participated in the study-and-work-in-Japan program organized by the non-profit organization Japan International Care Aid Organization (JICAO). For two years, starting in April 2006, he worked at a convalescent ward in a hospital in Tokyo while attending language school. Allan dreamt of acquiring the *kaigo fushishi* certificate and working in Japan. The director of the nursing service department at the hospital where Allan worked asserted: "Probably because Filipinos tend to have a stronger service-minded personality than the Japanese, he is always in great demand. There are many things that the Japanese staff can learn from him" (*Shimotsuke Shimbun* 2007b). Thus business groups may utilize the notion of "caring Filipinos" to maximize their own interest in capital accumulation. A brief illustration of the working conditions among "foreign" care labourers residing in Japan offers vital insights into the likely experience of Filipino migrant care workers.

Recently, increasing numbers of "foreigners" have been engaged in commodified care provision in Japan. This is reflected in the observation of one care facility representative, who points out that "foreign" workers are already making an important contribution to elder care in Japanese society (Yamazaki 2006, 8). Since the mid-2000s in particular, several labour-dispatch companies, such as IPS Tokyo Caregiving Academy, have launched courses for Filipinos residing in Japan – predominantly women who used to work as "entertainers" and who married (and, in many cases, subsequently divorced) Japanese men – to obtain the licence known as *kaigo herupa* (care helpers) level two. The latter is ranked below *kaigo fukushishi* and does not require that the exam be written in Japanese.[14] Kristine describes her experience of working as a *herupa:* "I completed school in 2004. Now, I have been working as a *herupa* for one year and eight months. The job is physically demanding. I have become tired. I work eight hours a day, including night shifts ... When I am told something, I listen to it obediently and learn about it. But once I understand what I need to do and how to do my work, if someone still tells me what to do and how to do it, I will speak back to that person." Her story underlines the importance of understanding political action not only as an activity associated with the formal conduct of governance but also as everyday social relations that involve the covert and overt (re)negotiation of power dynamics in contested spaces of work. Clearly, jobs performed by Filipina *herupa* are physically demanding. As low-rank care workers, Filipina *herupa* are frequently assigned to the night shift, where one attendant may be required to oversee twenty patients for sixteen to eighteen hours (Suzuki 2007, 374-75). When looking at the precarious employment conditions of "foreign" care workers living in Japan, one should pay heed to how the social spaces of work are produced in the everyday lives of Filipino care labourers who enter Japan through the JPEPA.

Under the JPEPA, the Japanese government issues *tokutei katsudo* (designated activity) visas to Filipino *kaigo fukushishi* candidates. During their four-year training period, these Filipinos are supposed to receive the same remuneration as their Japanese counterparts, be protected by Japanese labour law, and be covered by the Japanese insurance system (MHLW 2006). However, in Japan, the accelerated commodification of care labour following the implementation of LTCI, along with the cuts to nursing-care benefits, has depreciated the position of care work, rendering it feminized and socially undesirable. Poor employment conditions are reflected in the average annual incomes of *kaigo fukushishi*: 3.15 million yen for men and 2.81 million yen for women, which are much lower than the national average of 4.52 million yen (*Yomiuri Shimbun* 2007). The earnings of non-licensed care workers are even lower. A survey conducted by the Care Work Foundation reveals that Japanese care labourers are dissatisfied with their low wages, especially given the physical and mental demands of their work (Takagi 2006, 56-57). Thus, the policy of "same labour, same pay" for Filipino candidates, especially those without their Japanese certificate, only guarantees that they will receive the lowest remuneration within an already low-paid care labour market. The conditions of the JPEPA also restrict where these Filipino care workers may practise: even after passing the *kaigo fukushishi* examination, they can only work at care institutions.

Once these Filipino candidates enter the spaces of caregiving jobs in Japan, one of the most difficult barriers that they encounter is language. In the medical field, it is essential for workers not only to record the conditions of the patients and the content of the services in Japanese but also to comprehend them. As Takaki Kojima at the IPS Tokyo Caregiving Academy points out: "Because of the language limitations among the Filipino caregivers, the employers have asked them to do the jobs, such as excretion disposal, which the Japanese workers often do not want to do. This kind of problem happens frequently."[15] If Filipino care workers receive discriminatory job allocations even after their initial employment period, this will create class stratification based on race and nationality. This will reduce various issues of discriminatory relations in the workplace to differences of nationality, which may give rise to complicated disputes between labour and management (Asato 2007, 43).

Filipino care labourers coming to Japan under the JPEPA may also undergo "a painfully excruciating experience" of "social downward mobility" (Parreñas 2001b, 1132). Maria, who is currently carrying out OJT at TPV with the intention of working in Japan, notes: "Based upon my experience of taking care of the Japanese elderly, they are kind and polite ... But not all [of them are]. A few of the Japanese treat us at a very low level. Our job here is to take care of the elderly, including [doing their] household chores. So, their image of us is very low. They do not think of us as working here as professional caregivers. Some of them treat us like maids." Like Maria, Filipino care workers entering Japan have undertaken caregiver training and have obtained Philippine licences, but they will only be considered as *kaigo fukushishi* candidates whose purpose is to assist Japanese-certified care workers. Since many Filipinos leave their professional jobs in the Philippines to seek overseas employment, this non-recognition of their professional qualifications as care workers contributes to their underemployment and downward mobility. These distressing experiences of "contradictory class mobility" (Parreñas 2001a) among Filipino care workers may be exacerbated by racial discrimination towards, and scapegoating of, "foreigners."[16]

The Social Spaces of Leisure, Filipina-as-Entertainer Prejudice, and Political Rights

The survey conducted by the Care Work Foundation depicts how workers in the elder-care sector in Japan suffer from precarious employment (Takagi 2006). It reveals that, although more than 90 percent of its respondents note that they are entitled to annual paid holidays, approximately 40 percent of them cannot obtain days off when they want them. Based on these findings, Hiroshi Takagi (2006, 57) suggests that elder-care work in Japan is being sustained by the "self-sacrifice" of care workers. Being employed as low-rank labour, Filipino care workers are required to exhibit dedication that borders on self-sacrifice. What possibilities and difficulties do these conditions pose for Filipino care workers in their efforts to organize to contest discrimination in Japan? Some insight may be found by investigating the social spaces of leisure and political rights available to these labourers.

Whereas the political rights of "foreign" migrant workers in Japan are highly limited due to the fact that they lack both national and local suffrage (Kibe 2006), in the field of care provisioning, Filipino *herupa* have organized substantial alliances to challenge the discrimination they encounter in

Japan. For instance, in 2006, one group of certified *kaigo herupa* Filipinas founded the Licensed Filipino Caregivers Association in Japan (LFCAJ), which has a current enrolment of 170 Filipinas.[17] Based upon its motto, "to give care unbounded by race and country," the LFCAJ aims not only to foster close relationships with Japanese government authorities, educational organizations, and the care industry in order to improve the working conditions of Filipino care workers but also to represent Filipina caregivers to Japanese society. Its members have constructed social communication networks to tackle the problems that they encounter at work as well as to exchange job information.

For the many Filipinas residing in Japan who used to be nightclub "entertainers," care labour is recognized as a "socially respectable job" (Suzuki 2007, 374). Joselyn, a *herupa* licence holder and LFCAJ member, comments:

> The feedback from my children changed once I started studying for caregiving and my work changed ... During the night, I used to work, so I could not stay with my children, but now I can stay with them ... I was so surprised that my children boasted about me to their teachers at school, saying, "My mother's work is very hard." The reactions of the people at the City Hall have changed as well. When I say that my occupation is caregiver, they say, "That is impressive!" I was happy since, until now, nobody admired me in Japan.

For these Filipinas, many of whom, like Joselyn, are divorced single mothers, elder-care work is a means not only of transcending their negative image as "entertainers" but also of securing stable incomes. More strikingly, Joselyn notes: "Based upon my ... experience [in] care labour, I want to provide support for the Filipino care workers who will come to work in Japan in the future." In fact, since its inception, the LFCAJ has attempted to create support mechanisms for the Filipino care workers who will come to Japan under the JPEPA, especially with regard to the linguistic-cultural barriers they will face. Nevertheless, as Suzuki (2007, 376) writes, although it is seemingly imperative for the "resident and incoming Filipinos ... to create working relationships with each other in order to effectively monitor the terms and conditions of work," doing so may not be easy.

Jane, a Philippine-certified caregiver who is undertaking OJT at TPV to prepare herself for working at Japanese care institutions, comments: "In dealing with nurses and other staff in Japan, we may face discrimination because they may think that Filipino girls are only [involved] in the entertainment business. It may be difficult to deal with them because of this discriminatory perspective ... [In order to transcend this bias among Japanese colleagues], we will do our best to prove that not all Filipino girls are entertainers." One of the Japanese nonprofit organizations promoting the acceptance of Filipino care workers emphasizes the importance of forming a mutual aid mechanism only among Filipino caregivers coming to Japan under the JPEPA – separate from resident Filipino *herupa* – to prevent the former from being associated with "sex workers."[18] This endeavour, while illustrating the widespread stigmatization of Filipino women in Japanese society, further reinforces it by constructing differentiation and hierarchy among Filipino care workers. In other words, the introduction of Filipino labour into Japan's care facilities requires changes in the thinking of both Filipinos and Japanese in order to overcome the sexist, classist, and racist representation of Filipino women. Such shifts not only allow incoming Filipinos to collaborate with experienced Filipino care labourers in dealing with the everyday struggle of working and living in Japan but also facilitate the incorporation of culturally/ethnically different "others," who, as new members of Japanese society, sustain the process of reproducing the social relations of (re)production.

Conclusion

Within the context of intensified globalization, the neoliberal restructuring of the social relations of (re)production has not only pushed capitalist norms deeper into the practices of social reproduction but, through the transnational migration of care workers, has also contributed to the international division of reproductive labour. This chapter focuses on the introduction of Filipino care workers into Japan under the JPEPA, demonstrating that the transnational migration of this commodified labour leads to a hierarchical regime of social reproduction structured along the lines of nationality, class, ethnicity, race, and gender. More specifically, it highlights the way state policy shifts towards the neoliberal governance of social (re)production have facilitated the currently emerging global division of reproductive labour through (1) the commodification of care work and (2) the constitution of migrant care workers as potentially cheap, flexible, and disposable racialized and gendered subjects. It also illuminates the everyday struggles, contestations, and negotiations of Filipino care workers who come to Japan. This analysis of the practices of Filipino care labourers not only exposes how their social, economic, and political rights may be limited but also suggests how, as political agents, they might challenge this.

The JPEPA itself forces Filipino care workers to undergo extensive training and examination, with no guarantee that they will be permitted to stay in Japan. And this violates their human rights and security. As this chapter shows, "foreign" immigrants, such as resident Filipino *herupa*, maintain the current Japanese elder-care system by working at the bottom of Japan's care labour market. Furthermore, there is the critical, but not widely discussed, issue of how to ensure the provision of care for the elderly Korean-Japanese – most of whom are not protected under LTCI, which is restricted to pension recipients (Kawano 2007; K. Lee 2007). It is thus imperative to recognize that the introduction of Filipino and other immigrant care labour to Japan is not a "new" issue; rather, it is part of Japan's effort to cultivate a system of "multiethnic/multicultural" elder-care provision. To facilitate this process, as Yoshiko Kuba (2007, iv) puts it: "The efforts to improve the working conditions of care workers and the 'quality of care' must be discussed in conjunction with the exploration of how to create Japan's social welfare regime by promoting 'social inclusions' of Korean-Japanese, *Nikkeijin* and diversified ethnic groups."

PART 2

Transnational Influence of Care Discourses

4 Transnationalizing (Child) Care Policy
The OECD and the World Bank

RIANNE MAHON

Much of the work on the transnationalization of care has focused on global care chains, discussed in previous chapters. Yet, the transnationalization of care also involves the elaboration and global transmission of social policy discourses. International organizations (IOs) such as the Organization for Economic Cooperation and Development (OECD) and the World Bank have played an important part in this, along with international non-governmental organizations (INGOs) like the Bernard van Leer Foundation, the Aga Khan Foundation, and, in Eastern Europe, the Soros Foundation. The work of the major international organizations is also supported by transnational knowledge networks, such as the Consultative Group on Early Childhood Care and Development. This chapter focuses on the role played by the OECD and the World Bank in putting early child education and care (ECEC) on policy agendas around the world.[1]

Although the OECD and the World Bank are often (rightly) associated with the promotion of neoliberal globalization, a closer examination of their policy discourses suggests that they have gone beyond counselling the brute neoliberal prescription of welfare cuts and structural adjustment. As part of their broader push for "social investment" (Jenson 2008), they have become advocates of public investment in child care/child development programs. This does not mean that they have abandoned the broader globalization project; rather, investing in children has come to be seen as a critical component of that project.

Somewhat ironically, given that globalization has meant the intensified export of carers from South to North, ECEC is advocated not only for OECD countries but also for the global South. Both versions of the ECEC discourse aim at the modification of postwar regimes, from the goal of greater equality in the here-and-now to equality of opportunity over the life course. Both also reflect the impact of global political developments in the name of gender equality and the rights of the child. At the same time, they differ in important respects. The dominant discourse directed at the South by the World Bank draws especially on the American social policy model, emphasizing provision through the market. It might be considered "neoliberalism plus" in that it integrates elements of social liberalism, such as Nobel prize winner Amartya Sen's emphasis on developing capabilities, into a residual social policy discourse refashioned to meet the demands of economic globalization. In contrast, the discourse directed at OECD member states exhibits the stronger influence of Western European, especially Scandinavian, experience.

This chapter examines how the main international organizations dealing with social policy have framed their arguments for child care, including the scientific and normative knowledge bases of their truth claims. International organizations are involved in policy learning in response to ideas travelling through the transnational discourse communities of which they form a part. The first sections locate the 1990s discovery of investing in children within its broader political and intellectual context. The next section analyzes two key OECD reports that call for increased investment in ECEC in the global North. The discussion then turns to discourses directed towards the South, focusing on the early childhood development discourses articulated by the World Bank.

Political Context(s) of Discovery

The promotion of ECEC at international scales is not entirely new. There is some evidence of efforts to promote preschool education in the early postwar years (Kamerman 2006). In the 1960s, the United Nations Educational, Scientific and Cultural Organization (UNESCO) began to collect data on preschools, and, in 1965, the United Nations Children's Fund's (UNICEF's) executive board recognized the period of one to six years as a "crucial missing link" in human growth and development (Myers 1991). Preschool was still considered a luxury, to be pondered only after primary and secondary education were available for all. The World Bank's interest in investment in human capital was confined to secondary and vocational education (Jones and Coleman 2005, 106). In 1972, UNESCO began to fund seminars on ECEC, but its 1974 conference on education for children from zero to six took a defensive tone, stressing that preschool would not harm the child's creativity (Kamerman 2006). In the same year, UNICEF's *Report on the Young Child* rejected preschool education in favour of improved maternal care (Myers 1991, 8-9), while the World Bank concluded that investment in preschool "could not be justified" (Kamerman 2006, 8).

Even while these IOs remained, at best, ambivalent, the OECD began to reflect on ECEC. Its perspective was clearly marked by the 1970s push for gender equality as well as by the care needs associated with women's rising labour force participation. The first report of the newly formed working party on the role of women in the economy (ROWITE) focused on *The Care of Children of Working Parents* (OECD 1974). Gender equality was the primary normative lens through which it viewed ECEC. Yet children's needs also figured in the calculus, perhaps because the OECD's Centre for Research and Education (CERI) was simultaneously engaged in studying ECEC. Exchange between these two units helps to account for the emergence of the concept of ECEC or policies to link preschool education and day care, which, until then, had been treated as two separate spheres. In contrast to some of the later studies, these OECD studies also recognized that ECEC only formed part of the equality puzzle (Mahon 2009).

Many of the points made in the OECD studies would reappear in the policy discourses of various international organizations twenty-five years later. In the 1980s, however, with the ascendancy of neoliberalism, ECEC largely disappeared from the IOs' agendas. In the North, this entailed promoting social expenditure cuts. In the South – and, later, countries of the former Soviet Bloc, many of which had had publicly financed child care – the World Bank and the International Monetary Fund (IMF) made access to financial assistance conditional upon the adoption of austere structural adjustment packages.

There was, of course, resistance to "roll-back" neoliberalism, and not only at the grassroots level. Some international organizations entered the fray, led by UNICEF under the banner of adjustment with a human face. Consistent with its mandate, UNICEF emphasized the cost of adjustment for young children, "the most vulnerable section of the population, yet also the one more important for the future of the country" (Jolly 1991, 1810). UNICEF thus helped to create a space for the "social investment paradigm," focused on children (Jenson 2008). Yet, UNICEF did not challenge the need for adjustment. While it called for the preservation of a minimum level of nutrition, income, and services, it also sanctioned the "serious restructuring" of social services to achieve the maximum cost-effectiveness and internal efficiency, and pointed to the possibility of a "more creative reliance on community action and the informal sector" (Jolly 1991, 1810). Furthermore, it conceded the need to scale back existing welfare regimes, while arguing for programs targeting the poorest – especially children.

At the Eighteenth World Conference of the Society for International Development in 1985, Jolly presented "Adjustment with a Human Face" to an audience that included World Bank representatives. In light of the ensuing debates, "some in the World Bank, such as Alan Berg and Paul Isenman, subsequently used the occasion to encourage broader thinking, circulating copies of *Adjustment with a Human Face* to colleagues within the World Bank and to others outside" (Jolly 1991, 1814). Berg was one of the Bank officials who would later support the World Bank's embrace of investment in children.

The focus on young children was given added impetus by the 1989 Convention on the Rights of the Child. Although the committee did not take up the issue of ECEC until 2005, the widespread ratification of the convention added a potentially important rights basis to UNICEF's case for investment in children. In addition, the 1990 World Declaration on Education for All (EFA) recognized that learning begins at birth, while the subsequent EFA Framework of Action (2000) made "expanding and improving comprehensive early childhood care and education, especially for the most vulnerable and disadvantaged children," its first goal. The 1990 World Summit for Children similarly focused a spotlight on children's right to survival, protection, and development.

The Convention on the Rights of the Child introduced the concept of rights to the discourse on ECEC, helping to bring about a shift from the 1980s focus on needs (Myers 2000, 25). Such a rights orientation fit well with UNESCO's discourse, especially during the 1980s (Jones and Coleman 2005, 77). The dominant discourse, however, continued to emphasize needs, although the concept was broadened to include child development, in part as a result of the work of the then newly formed Consultative Group on Early Childhood Care and Development. One of the key figures associated with the Consultative Group, Robert G. Myers (1987), authored an important report on early child development for the World Bank. As a result, the IOs' agenda was reframed from child survival = reduction in child mortality to survival = a process "of change in which the child learns to handle ever more complex levels of moving, thinking, feeling and relating to others"

(Myers 1991, 19). It was interpreted, however, in a manner consistent with UNICEF's adjustment-with-a-human-face discourse. The early childhood development and care goal was thus defined as "expansion of early childhood care and development activities, *including family and community interventions, especially for poor, disadvantaged and disabled children*" (Myers 2000, 4 [emphasis added]). Thus, the emergent discourse favoured programs targeting poor, disadvantaged and disabled children and envisaged an important role for (cheaper) family and community interventions.

While the forging of an ECEC transnational discourse community focused attention on child development, the emergence of a transnational women's movement, aided by the UN Decade for Women (1976-85), injected a gender dimension into the social investment discourse (Friedman 2003; Kardam 2004). Here again, UNICEF contributed by demonstrating that "the adjustment process typically added burdens to women in their roles as household managers and parents while often reducing the time and finance available to support them in these roles" (Jolly 1991, 1817). Gender equity would also figure in the ECEC discourse of the World Bank, but less as a matter of equality between men and women than as a means for levelling the playing field between boys and girls with regard to access to education.

Truth Claims

Scientific truth claims have also influenced the IO's ECEC discourses. One strand of research that has been particularly influential in persuading the World Bank of the importance of the very early years (zero to three) came from the field of neuroscience. In the 1990s, major American foundations began to distil the policy implications of this research. Thus the Carnegie-sponsored study, *Starting Points* (Carnegie Task Force on Meeting the Needs of Young Children 1994), focused attention on the quiet crisis affecting American children under three due to inadequate prenatal care, the rising number of lone parents, the substandard daycare available to the adult worker family, and poverty. The study highlighted the critical prenatal development of the human brain, noting its continued rapid development in the first year, and emphasized the environmental impact on the way the brain is wired. This research brought the early years to a "lifelong learning" agenda.

While some find in this research a rationale for public support for ECEC for all, these findings have been primarily interpreted as justification for (1) a turn from programs for older workers – even tertiary education – to children and youth, and (2) ECEC programs targeting the disadvantaged. This is supported by the contributions of economists like J.J. Heckman (1999, 39) of the University of Chicago, whose cost-benefit analyses of human capital formation at different stages of the lifecycle strongly favour investment in the young over investment in adults.

While Heckman made the utilitarian case for early child development, the work of Amartya Sen on "human capabilities" helped to marshal ethical claims in support of similar programs. Drawing out the implications of his work for ECEC, Sen (2003, 78) argued that "the capabilities that adults enjoy are deeply conditional on their experiences as children" and that "a securely preparatory childhood can augment our skill in living a good life." Sen's capabilities approach draws on an important strand of social liberalism that harks back to John Stuart Mill, who envisaged a positive role for governments in enabling individuals to develop to their full potential. While in the previous era, social liberalism was interpreted as support for the Keynesian-welfare state, in the discourses of IOs like the World Bank, the capabilities approach became part of adjustment with a human face. Thus, structural adjustment measures need to be supplemented with investment in early child development to break the intergenerational poverty cycle.

Other social scientists have contributed to the ECEC rationale. Gøsta Esping-Andersen (1999) cast his argument for ECEC as part of a broader project of welfare redesign. Echoing other critiques of Western European social insurance-based systems, Esping-Andersen was especially critical of the conservative-corporatist regimes of Western Europe for clinging to social programs targeted at the male breadwinner family instead of focusing on the needs of the time-pressed dual-earner family with young children. Although he took his inspiration from the Nordic social policy model, he drew back from recommending its extension to other advanced countries, content to make a pitch for some form of investment in ECEC. Esping-Andersen's work influenced the social policy paradigm that began to take shape in the OECD's Directorate for Employment, Labour and Social Affairs (DELSA). This, in turn, helped to pave the way for the *Babies and Bosses* study to be discussed below.

The World Bank's critique of European social insurance-based systems extends to the social security regimes of certain Latin American and Asian countries, which it sees as favouring insiders at the expense of the real poor. The Bank is also critical of universal programs. Thus, it argues that "governments do not tap the willingness of households to contribute resources directly to education"; "current financial arrangements result in a misallocation, with heavy subsidization of higher education at the expense of primary"; and resources in schools "are not used as efficiently as they might be," a problem "reinforced by lack of competition among schools" (Jones and Coleman 2005, 119). Similar arguments appear in the World Bank's counsel on investment in ECEC.

The policy discourses emanating from these sources have not gone unchallenged. In the decade prior to Esping-Andersen and colleagues' (2002) report to the president of the European Union, the European Commission had established its Childcare Network under the direction of Peter Moss, who was committed to an egalitarian vision of ECEC. The network began to develop a blueprint for a European ECEC strategy and to forge an alternative ECEC discourse community that found its inspiration in the Nordic and Reggio-Emilia ECEC approaches. Both emphasize the importance of child development, while the Nordic model adds strong public support to the promotion of gender equality. The network thus developed a conception of quality quite different from the dominant "developmentally appropriate practice" that dominates the US discourse.

Dahlberg and Moss (2008) highlight important differences between the discourse emanating from this network and the dominant Anglo-American one:

1 Whereas the dominant Anglo-American discourse stresses a future oriented instrumental rationality (human capital in the making), the alternative stresses an "ethics of encounter" (child in the here and now)
2 Whereas the first stresses the application of techniques to achieve pre-determined outcomes, the second stresses a plurality of possibilities – the child as co-constructor of knowledge and an active citizen
3 Whereas quality for the first measures the extent to which services conform to externally prescribed norms, a technology of normalisation, for the latter, quality develops in an open-ended, dialogical way.

While the European Commission officially disbanded its Childcare Network in the mid-1990s, it has remained alive as an egalitarian segment in the ECEC transnational discourse community and has grown in scale, helped, in part, by another OECD thematic study: *Starting Strong*.

ECEC for OECD Countries: Gender Equality and Children's Rights

The OECD's ECEC studies highlight its importance as a service to the "time-pressed" adult-earner family. There are, however, important differences – as, for example, between *Babies and Bosses* (OECD 2005) and *Starting Strong*

(OECD 2006) – in the way the argument was framed, the transnational discourse communities involved, and their impact on the organizational discourses of the two OECD directorates involved. The *Babies* study fit DELSA's social investment discourse and operated through the channels provided by the Working Party on Social Policy of the Employment, Labour and Social Affairs Committee, which brings together leading social policy officials from the member countries. This is not to suggest that learning did not occur. The *Babies* team developed a greater appreciation of the gender equality dimension, and these lessons have been institutionalized in the OECD's new family database, making possible ongoing comparison of member country performance in this area. The team did not, however, seek to create a transnational discourse community that went beyond the official Working Party network, nor did it connect with the ECEC transnational discourse community.

To head *Starting Strong*, the Education Directorate engaged an outside expert who was linked to the egalitarian ECEC discourse community. John Bennett had been involved in the UN Committee on the Rights of the Child while being in charge of UNESCO's Child and Youth Program. Although the *Starting Strong* team drew on the OECD's official network of experts, it also worked in such a way as to strengthen the egalitarian wing of this transnational community. Those involved hoped to sustain this network and thus to transform the Education Directorate's CEC discourse.

The *Babies* study, launched in 2001 and concluded in 2005, produced a number of background papers exploring various issues and collected data on various countries. DELSA's organizational discourse, which had incorporated a new conception of social policy in the 1990s, helped to frame *Babies* research.

DELSA's social policy discourse did not query the core goals of economic globalization and the concomitant need for policy redesign. Where it differed from "adjustment with a human face" was in its main object – the adult-earner family. The main problem was not seen as (class) inequality, though that was clearly on the rise, as a recent (2008) OECD study documents, nor was it especially concerned about lone-parent families and the poverty to which their children are exposed. Rejecting a narrow "workfare" approach, DELSA focused on all adult-earner families and the resulting social policy challenges posed by the "new demands for services traditionally produced within the home, particularly those relating to the care of children and other dependent relatives, and an increasing need for policy directions that [would] facilitate a balance between work and family responsibilities" (OECD 1994, 10).

The ideas laid out in *New Orientation for Social Policy* (OECD 1994) and developed through in-house research and conferences provided the ideational framework for *Babies*. Consistent with DELSA's embrace of a social investment discourse, *Babies* carefully scrutinized tax and benefit policies to identify disincentives to women's labour market participation. It accepted that, if more women were working outside the home, then there would be increased need for public support for non-parental child care as, on their own, markets might not deliver the spaces needed at a price many parents could afford. Nevertheless, public-sector monopolies are to be avoided, while demand subsidies are preferred to investment on the supply side as the latter only benefit those able to obtain a place. More important, demand-side subsidies support a market for care, thus putting pressure on providers to keep costs down while meeting parental demand. *Babies* did not ignore issues of quality, but, in contrast to the dialogical conception of quality offered by the European Commission Childcare Network, it adopted a new public management approach that sees child-care providers as self-interested agents to be controlled by "quality assurance" programs, backed by the discipline of market forces.

Parental leave is also an important part of the new family-friendly policy, but long leaves are rejected as destructive of a mother's human capital. The *Babies* team initially assumed that it would be mothers who would take "parental" leave, but it began to stake out a gender equality stance on this issue such that, by the fourth volume, it was prepared to criticize Sweden – one of the countries that has pushed for shared leave in the interests of gender equality – for not going far enough (Mahon 2010b).

DELSA's recognition of the role child-care arrangements can play in promoting gender equality can be traced in part to the impact of the feminist expert – Janet Gornick – hired to develop a framework for the family database. The resulting database, in turn, established the foundation for future governance through surveillance on these issues. The new database includes many of the areas highlighted in the earlier ROWITE studies: pay gaps between full- and part-time workers, male and female earnings, distribution of working hours between men and women, the gender distribution of child-care leave, and a typology of child-care benefits, including quality indicators.

The gender equality lessons that might have been learned from the earlier ROWITE studies thus had to be learned anew by the OECD's social policy division. Yet, while ROWITE was in an OECD that was still committed to the Keynesian welfare state, *Babies*' learning occurred within an organizational discourse that embraced economic globalization and the macroeconomic "fundamentals" associated therewith. In this universe, however, there is a role for "good" social policies that encourage working-age women as well as men to remain active labour market participants. I elsewhere label this approach "inclusive liberalism" (Mahon 2006b).

Although ECEC formed only a part of the range of "family-friendly" measures considered in *Babies*, it was central to the work of *Starting Strong*. While the latter by no means ignored gender equality, it focused on the child, much as the World Bank has done. Unlike the Bank, *Starting Strong* rejected the "child-as-human-capital-in-the-making" perspective in favour of children as active citizens in the here and now. The final volume placed particular emphasis on the need to ensure that the "well-being, early development and learning [are placed] at the core of ECEC work, while respecting the child's agency and natural learning strategies" (OECD 2006).

Starting Strong also took a very different view of child-care staff than did *Babies*. Accordingly, it was critical of the "low recruitment and pay levels ... the lack of certification in early childhood pedagogy ... the feminisation of the workforce and the failure of pedagogical teams to reflect the diversity of the neighbourhoods they serve" found in many countries (OECD 2006, 17). *Starting Strong* paid particular attention to early child pedagogy, contrasting "school readiness" approaches to the social pedagogy approach that combines "care, upbringing and learning, without hierarchy" (OECD 2006, 59). In other words, "educating the educators" combined with democratic governance is the solution, not market discipline.

The emphasis on the child does not mean that adults were forgotten. In particular, in the final volume, *Starting Strong* underlined the need for both "gender equality" – women's right to equal treatment in work, equal pay for equal value, and equal opportunities for advancement and "gender equity" – "equal sharing of child rearing and domestic work" (OECD 2006, 30). *Starting Strong* also took up the issue of child poverty. Like *Babies* it recognized that child care is helped by strengthening family income, especially for lone parents, and it also saw a role for ECEC in preventing the intergenerational transmission of poverty. Unlike the World Bank, however, it recognized that ECEC could only be part of the solution to child poverty, which is rooted not in welfare dependency or poor parenting but in the underemployment of parents, income inequalities, and insufficient transfer payments (23).

While *Starting Strong* drew on the ideas generated by the egalitarian element of the transnational ECEC discourse community, it also worked to broaden and deepen the networks sustaining that community. Thus, it reached out to like-minded experts across the OECD, organizing several transnational workshops on particular themes and, on the occasion of the release of the two summary reports (2001 and 2006), two major conferences, strategically sited in Stockholm and Reggio Emilia, respectively. As the final volume noted: "this systematic exchange of ideas on policy issues and their implementation was helpful and allowed participants to establish their own 'critical friend' networks" (OECD 2006, 233). At the Reggio Emilia conference, participants agreed to establish a permanent network and to report to the Education Committee in order to ensure the incorporation of *Starting Strong*'s perspective on the Education Directorate's organizational discourse. Housed in Flemish-speaking Belgium *(Kind und Gezin)*, the network functioned independently for a couple of years. In April 2008, however, it was taken over by the Education and Training Policy Division, whose understanding of ECEC is more in line with the Education Directorate's official discourse.

Early Childhood Development as Poverty Reduction

The World Bank, UNICEF, and UNESCO are all involved in spreading the early childhood development message to the global South, flanked by an array of INGOs and networks of experts such as the Consultative Group. This section focuses on the World Bank. As Jones and Coleman (2005, 94) note, "the combination of its financing levels and the force with which it promotes its views help account for its emergence as the strongest player in the world of multilateral education." This holds true for ECEC. While, in the 1960s and 1970s, the World Bank focused on vocational education, by the 1990s, it had embraced early childhood development as part of its broader investing-in-people agenda. Now, "it regards itself as an important contributor to the debate about childhood; conversely it is lobbied by many organizations that regard it as a major player in the field" (Penn 2002, 122).

While the World Bank draws on some of the same discursive elements as does DELSA, the Bank's ECEC message is shaped by its poverty-centred organizational discourse. This, plus its clear bias in favour of American research, means that it focuses more on "early childhood development," drawing heavily on the scientific case for intervention in the early years, including prenatal care. ECEC is thus just one part of a package of measures targeting very young children who are poor. This is not to suggest that gender equality is ignored. Yet, the Bank's emphasis is on girl children as future workers and mothers, while adult women figure mainly as maternal agents to be enlisted in ensuring the development of the next generation. The role of the latter as workers, while not unimportant, is clearly secondary.

The reformulation of the World Bank's social policy discourse was directly affected by UNICEF's 1980s campaign for "adjustment with a human face," although mounting resistance to the Washington Consensus[2] provided the wider context. Some within the Bank were quick to seize the opportunity thus provided. Under the presidency of Barber Conable (1986-91), the Bank began to fashion its new Core Poverty Program (Hall 2007, 155). Initially focused on the need for residual social safety nets, the program was expanded to incorporate the message that "investment in human resources through health, education and population was good for growth" (ibid.). Like adjustment with a human face, the new organizational discourse did not imply a rejection of structural adjustment. This is clearly evident in two subsequent publications – *Investing in People* (World Bank 1995b) and *Building Human Capital for Better Lives* (World Bank 1995a).

Building Human Capital argued the importance of working on two fronts: "sound macroeconomic policies" to promote growth, complemented by human investment "so that people will have the skills and abilities to take advantage of those opportunities " (World Bank 1995a, 2). Investment in human capital aims to enable the poor and disadvantaged to participate in the liberalizing global economy (Psacharopoulos 1995, 2). Or, as *Investing in People* put it: "Investment in people implies striving to reach the point at which human capital investments no longer restrain growth or keep people in absolute poverty. Vital in this is equipping the poor to take advantage of the expanding opportunities that accompany growth" through "extending better health, nutrition and family planning to the poor" (World Bank 1995a, 24).

The Bank did not mean public investment in *all* people; rather, social expenditure should be restructured, eliminating subsidies for the elite. Thus, "Bank operations have rationalized post-secondary and higher education spending [which are seen primarily to benefit the advantaged] and attempted to redirect expenditures to primary education" (World Bank 1995a, 8).[3] Public expenditures should focus on the poor and disadvantaged.

Women are numbered among the disadvantaged, but with the focus on girls (human capital in the making) and mothers able to affect the quantity and quality of future human capital. Thus, *Building* cites "the impact of women's health and education on their childbearing decisions and the health and survival chances of their children, as well as their earning potential and employment opportunities" in making its case for "investing in women"

(Psacharopoulos 1995, 9). Traditional maternal practices rather than the structural factors behind poverty, exacerbated by adjustment policies, are blamed for child malnutrition. Thus, *Building* states: "Malnutrition of very young children rarely reflects a lack of food in the home. More often it is the product of feeding practices, child care practices and the health environment to which the child is exposed" (Psacharopoulos 1995, 31).

The new discourse retains the World Bank's earlier preference for privatization and "public-private partnerships." Like *Babies and Bosses*, *Investing in People* encourages the expansion of private provision in the name of greater efficiency, quality, and equity. Thus, "rather than supporting only government 'monopolies' as suppliers of education, the Bank is working with 'vouchers,' community-run schools, and other instruments ... to give families more choice ... or more voice" (World Bank 1995b, 8). The growth of private schools is also seen as an advantage as it would let the "elite," who can pay for their children's education, do so, thereby freeing spaces in public schools for poor children (World Bank 1995b, 11).

Thus, the World Bank's social investment discourse holds to the original neoliberal thrust of the Washington Consensus. At the same time, it concedes a role for the right kind of social policy – targeted programs to develop the capabilities of the poor, especially those of the next generation. While the Bank is prepared to offer financial support for such ventures, local governments are to free up revenue by disinvesting in universal programs seen primarily to benefit the "elite." As Deacon (2007, 40) notes, "the Bank's technical experts, who were very able to measure who received public services, were ill-informed about the political economy of welfare state building, which requires cross-class alliances in defence of public expenditure."

By the mid-1990s, early childhood development had clearly become part of the Bank's strategy, and its interpretation of the problem fit neatly into investing-in-people discourse. In fact, "multisectoral approaches to early childhood development" is the first of the next steps listed in *Building*.

In 1989, paediatrician Mary Eming Young was hired as a child development specialist within the Human Development Network – the Bank division most influenced by the social investment discourse described above. By 1992, ECD components had begun to appear in Bank educational projects, and a number of Bank country education strategy papers provided additional support from the field (Young 1995, 9). Since then, numerous studies have been commissioned, and the Bank has hosted two major international ECD conferences (in 1996 and 2000, respectively) and several regional conferences on ECD. It is also involved in several projects in partnership with other IOs and INGOs.

The World Bank's ECD research draws on information from the Bank's own projects in the field and input from the US "High/Scope" educational research foundation, UNICEF, the Inter-American Development Bank, USAID, Save the Children US, the Bernard van Leer Foundation, and the Aga Khan Foundation. Young's first public report (1995) refers to the Carnegie and Rand studies mentioned earlier, while later publications draw on Heckman's argument for the efficiency of investment in the early years. The Bank's first ECD conference was also held in conjunction with the Atlanta-based Task Force on Child Survival and Development (now the Center for Child Well-Being). Penn (2002, 123) is thus largely correct in criticizing Young's work for failing to "mention any developed country except the USA, even though there is considerable documentation from various European and Antipodean sources to suggest that conceptions of early childhood programmes in these countries may be very different."

These sources, filtered through the Bank's own "investing-in-people" lens, framed the case for ECD. Thus, the case for ECD drew heavily on neuroscience and behavioural science discoveries, while also relying on the notion of "developmentally appropriate practice." As the definition of ECD provided on the Bank's ECD home page notes: "All children progress through an identical sequence of physical, cognitive, and emotional growth and change. The ECD approach is based on the proven fact that young children respond best when caregivers use specific techniques designed to encourage and stimulate progress to the next level of development."[4] While developmentally appropriate practice was initially advanced as a counter to the "schoolification" of ECEC (Bennett 2008), Penn (2002, 125) underlines the liberal assumptions – the centrality of the individual, the need to encourage choice – that came to permeate the discourse.

In line with the American social model, the World Bank argues for a targeted approach to ECD in the name of "equity" and efficiency. Here it draws on the normative claims advanced by thinkers like Rawls and Sen as reflected in the following statement by one of Young's mentors: "A minimum notion of what constitutes 'social justice' would exclude any state in which some groups of children are deprived of having a reasonable chance to live a productive life just because they are born poor. Even societies that are unable, or unwilling, to provide a 'level playing field' ... may want to put policies in place that allow all who have reasonable talents and are willing to use them, a chance to enjoy at least a minimum level of well-being" (Van der Gaag and Tan 1998, 32). A corollary is that middle-class families should be expected "to contribute to the cost of their investment in the future of their children" (33). Thus, countries like Brazil err in investing scarce public dollars in universal preschool programs (Young 2002, 132).

The World Bank also commends less-expensive community-based programs and public-private partnerships that offer the additional benefit of employment opportunities for local women (Young 2002, 136). Thus *Investing in Children* argues:

> Mothers can be effective ECD providers in home-based programs, such as in Colombia and Bolivia. The women receive training and minimum assistance, on credit, to meet facility standards. They are "accredited" as eligible to provide day-care services. Such efforts enable providers to benefit from public subsidies while also participating in a competitive, choice-based system of ECD programs. In addition, they benefit parents by increasing the number and type of care options to choose from (e.g., based on convenience, proximity, flexibility of hours). By helping to create new providers locally, government helps consolidate the players, power, position, and perception of early child development, primarily at the local level. (Young 1995, 386-87)

Yet, such programs not only fail to provide genuine ECEC, they also feed into the growth of the informal sector, which the Bank's adjustment policies have done so much to promote (Beneria 2008).[5]

Conclusion

The lines of division between the OECD and the World Bank sketched above perhaps exaggerate the differences between the two policy discourses. Thus, the recent report by UNICEF's research division (Florence-based Innocenti), directed at OECD countries, draws on some of the same neuroscientific and economics research as does the Bank in making its argument that the current "child care transition" holds the potential for harm as well as for good. While the Innocenti study continues to favour universality, it follows the American/World Bank line in arguing that disadvantaged children should be given priority (9). It also advocates a mix of public and private provision, although here its position is not much different from that staked out in the OECD's *Babies* series.

The *Babies* discourse shares a number of elements with the Bank's, notably the emphasis on the macroeconomic realities essential to economic globalization and new public management's preference for private provision, including cheaper forms of child care, made in the name of choice. This supports Craig and Porter's (2004) argument that the post-Washington Consensus social policy discourses directed to the advanced capitalist countries as well as to the global South can both be described as inclusive liberalism. More broadly, none of these discourses takes up the challenge of incorporating a relational "ethics of care," although *Starting Strong* comes a lot closer to so doing. Yet, Williams (2001, 486) notes, "as the practices and values of care are becoming internationalized, arguments for a political ethics of care are as important among international policy-making bodies as they are among nation states."

Nevertheless, important differences remain. The World Bank and its networks draw their inspiration from the residual American social policy model, targeting the poor while leaving the rest to rely on markets and families. *Babies* and *Starting Strong* both reflect the influence of European social policy models embodying the principle of universality. Another critical difference is in the treatment of women. The Bank, departing from American practice, if not from the "family values" of the American New Right, still emphasizes women's (current and future) maternal role. In contrast, both OECD studies echo the European Union's commitment to women's equality with men in the labour market and the importance of shared parental leave.

How can we account for these differences? At one level, they reflect the particular organizational discourses through which each organization has come to see the world. Though both IOs can be seen as nodes in the ECEC transnational discourse community, the roles they play within this reflect the distinct organizational discourses filtering their selections from research conducted elsewhere. More broadly, geo-political location may have influenced their research strategies. That the Bank's social policy model bears a strong resemblance to the residualist American social policy model is not accidental. As Wade (2002, 318) notes: "The large majority of Bank economists have a postgraduate qualification from a North American university, whatever their nationality ... [t]he Bank's location in the heart of Washington ... plus the fact that its staff read US newspapers and watch American TV, plus the fact the English is the only language of business, mean that American pressures structure the very mindset with which most Bank staff promote development." In contrast, the OECD's headquarters are in Paris, the majority of member states are European, and Europeans constitute the majority of its professional staff. Jackson (2008) suggests that this has enabled the addition of social democratic ideas to the policy mix, especially with the victories of left governments in key European states during the latter half of the 1990s. In addition, there are strong connections between the European Commission and the OECD. The European Union is an active participant in many of its committees and has representation on the Ministerial Council. The two collaborate on various projects, although the OECD's longer research involvement around labour market and social policy issues and larger staff complement means that it is the European Commission that looks to the OECD rather than the reverse.

One final difference is the addressee. The World Bank focuses on the global South, which is to be admonished to follow the "best practices" of the advanced capitalist countries. As Rojas (2004, 97-98) suggests: "The power of aid stems from the way it represents the Third World as in need of government, converting recipient countries into subjects of intervention and donors into their natural rulers. Aid establishes a relation between donor and recipient regulated by the promise of transforming the recipient country." While the OECD is broadening its reach, its membership consists primarily of advanced capitalist countries. *Babies* and *Starting Strong* examine the policies and practices of these countries, taking as their exemplars European social models. When the OECD addresses the South, however, its tone changes: "even if it is possible to characterize the OECD in terms of its views on national social policy for *developed* countries as even-handed and concerned as much with universalism, public provision, and equity as with targeting and market efficiency, this is not always the case with regard to its view on social policy in a *development* context" (Deacon and Kaasch 2008, 236, emphasis in original). This is especially clear in the work of its Development Assistance Committee (Ruckert, 2008).

Moreover, neither the OECD nor the World Bank call for a fundamental rethinking of fiscal policies that impose severe constraints on social spending, nor do they challenge existing social structures at the global and national scales. Thus, while IOs' geo-political headquarters may leave a strong imprint on the social policy and child-care discourses they develop, these discourses also reflect, and help to reproduce, deeper inequalities between the North and the South.

5

Social Investment Policy in South Korea

ITO PENG

Since the beginning of the 2000s, the South Korean (hereafter Korean) government has taken on an explicit social investment strategy. The clearest example of this is the expansion of social care. Under the Roh Moo-hyun administration (2003-08), welfare support for the family and child care expanded, and long-term care insurance (LTCI) was introduced, universalizing care for the elderly. When the conservative government headed by President Lee Myung-bak took office in 2008, people initially feared that it would cut social spending and reverse the course of welfare expansion. Their fears proved unfounded. In fact, the current government has not only stayed on the same social policy track but has also made even more explicit its commitment to social investment by further expanding social welfare and social care. In this chapter I argue, first, that social-care policies introduced by the Korean government since 2003 represent a pragmatic response to multiple social and political pressures and, second, that Korean policy makers have adopted this course as a result of active policy learning and policy transfer. The Korean case thus offers a useful window on: (1) the nature of the social investment paradigm that is now widely adopted among OECD countries and (2) the process of international policy learning and transfer as well as policy change.

The first section of this chapter provides an overview of the literature on policy learning and transfer while the second examines social-care expansion in Korea since 2000. Although there has been significant expansion in both child and elder care, I focus on child-care and family-work reconciliation policies, highlighting the socio-economic and political factors that have influenced policy changes. In the third section, I reflect on the process of policy learning and policy change using the case of child care. I show how policy makers and other political actors in Korea used the available social policy models provided by international organizations such as the OECD and UNICEF to make the case for policy change and to develop new policy programs. While the process of policy learning and transfer may be fairly straightforward, the actual process of change is not so simple. As child-care policy reform illustrates, policy making remains a highly political process in Korea. I conclude by drawing out the implications for policy learning offered by the Korean case.

Policy Learning and Transfer

Ideas, cognitive paradigms, or taken-for-granted worldviews influence the way policy makers and political actors perceive and define social problems and, hence, consider policy solutions and alternatives (Campbell 2002, 2004). For example, in familialistic welfare states (such as Korea, Japan, Italy, and Spain), assumptions about the role of the family in providing individual welfare and care act as a powerful rationale for the state to relegate responsibility for social welfare to the family. Similarly, in many countries, the male breadwinner household model serves as a cognitive template in formulating policies to protect male employment, to support a family wage, and to defend the pension rights of full-time housewives. Once in place, such policies, in turn, shape cultural and ideational norms about family and gender relations, thus further reinforcing the existing system. In short, social policies are developed, on the one hand, through iterative processes between structure and institution and, on the other, through cognitive paradigms constructed by political actors as they engage in defining and solving problems.

New policy ideas are often generated and transmitted through the process of policy learning and transfer. Rose (1991a, 1991b), for example, argues that it is common for policy makers to look to policy experiences from other countries to draw lessons. Such international movement of social policy ideas and practices is important not only because it is an excellent source of policy learning and innovation but also because it can serve political purposes: international policy evidence is often used by domestic policy makers "to put an issue on an institutional agenda; to mollify political pressure; to emulate the actions of an exemplar; to optimize the search for the best policy; and to legitimate conclusions already reached" (Bennett 1991, 33). In addition, ideas obtained through policy learning can provide cognitive road maps for policy makers to puzzle out problems. For example, Blyth (2002) and Somers and Block (2005) argue that, in times of political crisis, ideas can help political actors to reformulate social problems and thus to identify new pathways to solving them.

What are the mechanisms of policy learning and transfer? Much attention has been paid to the roles of epistemic communities and policy networks or advocacy coalitions as the conduits for policy learning and policy transfer. Pointing to the significant transnational movement of social policy ideas between the United States and Europe, Haas (1992) and Hulme (2006) contend that epistemic communities, made up of knowledge-based experts with shared ideas based on "scientific knowledge," play an important role in the transfer of social policy models. Similarly, Sabatier and Jenkins-Smith (1993) claim that advocacy coalitions made up of networks of people with shared interests and common values can determine the direction of policy change through long-term interaction with policy makers.

In recent years, international organizations, such as the OECD, the UN, the IMF, and the World Bank have become increasingly important players within social policy epistemic communities. Not only do such think tanks play an important role in diffusing, transmitting, and advocating policy ideas within domestic and international arenas (Stone 2000) but international organizations such as the OECD have come to play a meditative role in policy innovation and translation (Mahon and McBride 2008). As a "purveyor of ideas," the OECD not only constructs and disseminates transnational research and policy ideas but also actively sets international policy norms by identifying problems and providing a range of "best practice" solutions. Mahon (this volume) also notes the intensification of global social policy discourses on ECEC and social investment policies as a part of the global policy harmonization effect of IOs and international NGOs.

Indeed, there is some evidence that modern nation-states and their policies are becoming increasingly isomorphic as they adopt "worldwide models" of behaviors and values, such as equality, human rights, and socioeconomic development. Some argue that these models are constructed and propagated by international organizations such as the UN. Meyer et al. (1997), for example, see national political actors and policy makers not so much as rational, self-directed actors engaged in constructing their own ideas but as "enactors of scripts" developed by international organizations. In this chapter, I argue that national political actors are not so scripted:

rather than simply "enacting scripts," they reinterpret, rewrite, and selectively adopt scripts to fit their national contexts.

In Korea, the idea of the developmental state, which saw social welfare as simply a subsidiary to economic development, was seriously challenged in the aftermath of the 1997 Asian economic crisis. While the shift seemed sudden, it reflected the impact of several deeper socio-economic changes that cast significant doubt on the validity of the existing welfare system and policies. Political and ideational contestations over the causes of, and solutions to, crises took place in both political and public arenas. Throughout the process, political actors drew on global policy ideas and networks to build their cases and to formulate alternative policy options. The outcome was a new perspective. Not only was the "pro-development" view (emphasizing economic development at all cost) eclipsed by the "pro-welfare" view (emphasizing economic redistribution as a policy priority), but policy makers and political actors also came to agree that the latter view, being in accordance with the ideational norms shared by other advanced industrialized nations, was the only reasonable one.

Social-Care Expansion in Korea

The Korean government has become the leading player in expanding family and child-care programs through legislation, financial incentives, and, in some cases, direct provision. Since 2004, significant efforts have been made to integrate ECE and ECC programs for children aged three to five and to create a "level playing field" by giving children from disadvantaged and low-income families priority access to ECEC programs. The ECEC reform plan includes fully integrated ECEC for preschool age children and the establishment of a free, universal, full-time ECEC program for five-year-olds (UNESCO 2006; Rhee 2007). Although the government has yet to achieve all its objectives, the recent ECEC policy reforms have led to a noticeable increase in the number of children in formal care: 37.7 percent enrolment rate for preschool age children, zero- to two-year-olds, in formal ECEC services in 2006 (up from 19.6 percent in 2004) and 79.8 percent for three- to five-year-olds (up from 59.5 percent during the same period) (OECD 2004; 2009).

Recent revisions to the Early Childhood Education Act and to the Child Care Act have led to the establishment of various interministerial and national-local ECEC-related committees tasked with expanding public support for child care and upgrading ECE and ECC certification requirements for service providers. The national government's ECE budget has more than doubled, from 334.7 billion won in 2002 to 886 billion won in 2006, while the ECC budget shot up from 479 billion won to 2,038 billion won. The introduction of sliding-scale financial support for ECEC in 2004 has led to a rapid increase in the number of children receiving child-care support fees, from 106,000 in 2002 to 563,000 in 2007 (Rhee 2007).[1] For children between the ages of three and twelve months, in 2007, 2.6 billion won was allotted for low-cost babysitting and night-time babysitting (*Chosun Daily* 2007).

In addition to child care, the 2001 Maternity Protection Act extended maternity leave from sixty to ninety days (at 100 percent wage replacement) and added an additional nine-month parental leave, thus enabling parents to take up to one year of leave. In 2004, to encourage parents to take parental leave, a flat-rate wage replacement of 300,000 won (approximately US$300) per month was added to the remaining nine months of parental leave. The rate was raised to 400,000 won in 2006 and to 500,000 won in 2007. The government further extended the period of parental leave from one to three years for public servants in 2006 (Korea Net 2006) and introduced a three-day paternity leave in 2008. Affirmative action legislation for working women was introduced in 2006 (Choi 2008). Within the National Basic Livelihood Security Program (social welfare), self-reliance support programs were implemented to help recipients, particularly lone mothers, get paid employment.[2] Between 2005 and 2006, the government also increased program support for single-parent families by about 150 percent.

There are several factors behind these policy changes. The first involves structural and normative transformations, including changes in household and marriage structure, fertility patterns, and ideas about gender relations. Between 1980 and 2006, the average Korean household size declined from 4.5 to 3.0. This reflects a drop in fertility (from 2.83 in 1980 to 1.13 in 2006) and an increase in the proportion of single-person households (KWDI 2008). The traditional pattern of intergenerational support has also weakened, as the proportion of people over the age of sixty living with their adult children declined (from 80 percent to 39 percent between 1981 and 2006). At the same time, the proportion of Korean women over the age of twenty-five with postsecondary education rose from 5.2 percent (1985) to 25.4 percent (2005), and the labour force participation rate of married women increased from 44.7 percent in 1985 to 51.3 percent in 2007 (KWDI 2008). Over the last two decades, the marriage age has risen, for Korean men, from 27.8 to 31.4, and for women, from 24.8 to 28.3 (KWDI 2008). Public opinion surveys also show that the majority of Koreans believe women should continue to work after marriage and/or childbirth (Na and Moon 2003; NSOK 2002).

In short, Korean society has undergone a rapid transformation over the last few decades. These changes have, in turn, led to new social and economic issues, including demographic aging, elder- and child-care needs, labour shortages, and increased public expectations about gender equality – all directly pointing to a need for policy change.

Second, Korea also experienced two critical political economic changes during the last couple of decades: political democratization in 1988 and the Asian economic crisis in 1997. Political democratization brought in competitive electoral politics and gave labour the right to form autonomous unions and to strike. The resulting combination of increased labour activism, rigid labour laws, and positive economic growth gave rise to rapid wage escalation, which, in turn, made the Korean economy increasingly uncompetitive, particularly against other newly industrializing Asian economies. The Korean government thus came under pressure from employers and economic policy bureaucrats to control wages and to deregulate the labour market. Their views gained added force when Korea joined the WTO in 1995 and the OECD in 1996 as, at that time, both organizations strongly supported increased labour market deregulation. With the Asian economic crisis of 1997, the Korean government was given IMF economic bailout conditions, which included an overhaul of the labour market.

The 1997 economic crisis brought about not only economic disruptions but also a political change, and, with this, changes in social policy. In response to IMF conditions, the newly elected left-of-centre Kim Dae-jung government (1998-2003) forged a state-business-labour tripartite social pact that exchanged employment deregulation for welfare state expansion. The result was huge worker layoffs, forced retirements, the replacement of regular with non-regular employees, and a rise in income inequality and poverty. At the same time, the government expanded social security and welfare provisions, such as employment insurance, national pensions, and the National Basic Livelihood Support Program, in order to offset the impacts of labour market deregulation. Social spending as a percent of GDP rose from about 3 percent in 1996 to 10 percent in 1999. This was, however, not enough to counter the worsening socio-economic situation. The Korean economy remained sluggish after the crisis, reinforcing the idea that Korea's high economic growth era had come to an end.

The Asian economic crisis exposed the deep integration of the Korean economy with the global economy, and it also marked the end of Korea's golden age (marked by state-led, export-led industrialization and rapid economic development) and a shift towards the postindustrial socio-economic phase. By the beginning of the new millennium, all these socio-economic and political factors had come together, creating massive and multiple pressures on the government to come up with a new policy vision.

Political Economy of Policy Change since 2000: Policy Imperatives and Policy Learning

The Roh Moo-hyun government, which took office in 2003, was saddled with multiple problems. In addition to the low economic growth rate, rising income inequality, and poverty, the total fertility rate continued to decline, raising concerns about demographic aging and care needs as well as labour shortages. To make matters worse, the new government's disappointing economic performance led the public and the media to repudiate the president. The government needed a new policy vision to maintain public support. In 2004, Roh Moo-hyun created several presidential commissions, including the Commission on Social Inclusion (to address the issues of poverty and income disparity); the Commission on Aging Society and Population Policy (to develop policies to deal with fertility decline and demographic aging); and the Commission on Policy Planning (to develop medium- and long-term policy strategies). All three commissions agreed that government policy should give priority to families and children. Their combined efforts were synthesized in the social and economic policy blueprint known as *Vision 2030* (Ministry of Planning and Budget 2007), which set the objective of raising the national per capita income to US$49,000 (from the 2006 level of US$14,000) and total social spending to 21 percent of GDP (from the 2007 level of 8.6 percent) by 2030. More important, *Vision 2030* framed the new policy goals in relation to a new paradigm based on social investment in human capital and the creation of a virtuous circle of positive returns between economic growth and social welfare development (Y. Kim 2007). In particular, it targeted social welfare expansion in areas of child and elder care as the "growth engine" for economic development (H. Lee 2007).[3]

Social investment was hailed as the symbol of the Roh government's new policy paradigm, a radical departure from the previous political regimes. In his keynote address, "Learning from Korea: Innovative Social Investment Strategies for Future Generations," which he gave to American policy makers and policy experts at the New America Foundation in Washington, DC, in

March 2007, Minister of Health and Welfare Simin Rhyu highlighted his government's new policy direction:

> The Ministry of Health and Welfare [of Korea] decided to go for a paradigm shift: encouraging self-development of all citizens, especially those who are underprivileged, and offering equal opportunities ... The traditional idea of welfare tends to be "this or that" kind of dichotomy. So, it's growth or distribution, development or welfare. However, we came to the conclusion that the state's investment in individuals should expand to enable each and everyone to develop their capacities and ensure everyone is given equal opportunities, by devising a system where economic growth and social policies supplement each other. Our priority is investment in human capital, especially children and the elderly, investment in health and investment in after-retirement life. (Rhyu 2007, 2-3)

Korea's social investment paradigm reflects a combination of cumulative policy learning and policy rethink within the Roh government. Korean policy makers and researchers had been examining Western and Japanese social policy models as early as the 1960s (Peng 2008; Peng and Wong 2008). Global social policy learning intensified after political democratization, especially after 1996, when Korea was admitted to the OECD. For a newly industrialized nation such as Korea, the accession to the OECD meant acceptance into the family of developed industrialized nations. This was a pledge of good international standing, a mark of the country's economic and social progress. Yet, it also put pressure on Korea to achieve social policy standards that were in line with those of other industrialized nations. Korean policy makers therefore needed to attend to the OECD and its cognate international organizations' social policy framework and the international discourse on social policy reforms.

The shift in Korea's social policy paradigm towards social investment came shortly after its entry into the OECD. The turn to investing in children came from a combination of (1) standards and expectations set by international organizations and (2) domestic policy actors who had come to believe in the importance of achieving those targets. In 1996, the Presidential Commission on Education Reform was established to realign the country's ECE with international standards. Many ECE experts saw this as an opportunity to streamline Korea's parallel track systems of ECE and ECC. Using UNESCO's recommendations, the commission argued for integrated full-day ECEC programs for three- to five-year-olds. In 1997, the commission tabled but failed to pass ECE reform legislation through a member's bill in Parliament. It tried three more times (in 1999, 2001, and 2003), but each time it failed to make progress.

The commission's ECE reform bill was drafted and tabled by National Assembly members largely in response to pressure from public kindergartens and ECE experts (UNESCO 2003). It failed to pass, in part, because they failed to consult with other stakeholders, particularly the child-care and private ECE sectors, which had significant vested interests in protecting the existing parallel system of child-care services and early child education as well as a market niche for private ECE. Fearing that the bill would result in the Ministry of Education and Human Resource Development's (MOEHRD) taking over ECEC, and thus threatening their businesses, child-care service providers (public and private child-care centres and child-care workers) and "Haekwons,"[4] together forming a much larger employer and labour group than did the kindergarten and ECE service sector, put up a fierce fight against the reform bill. The Ministry of Health and Welfare was also unwilling to go along with the ECE reform proposal as it would likely have meant the loss of its jurisdiction over child care for three- to five-year olds. Second, the advocates of the ECE reform bill also failed to make a clear distinction between their reform bill and the education reform bill that MOEHRD was developing at the time. As a result, people paid little attention to ECE reform, thinking that it was a small part of the larger educational reform being formulated by MOEHRD (Rhee et al. 2008).

The Presidential Commission on Education Reform and those who supported the ECE reform, however, remained resolute. Many came out of the experience with an understanding that they needed to reframe the bill and to raise it again at a different time. In an interview with the *UNESCO Courier* in 2003, Jung Na, senior researcher at the Korea Education Development Institute, and the architect of the ECE reform bill, argued that, instrumentalist objectives notwithstanding, achieving ECE reform was a matter of time, part of a natural policy progression as the country moved from a developing to a developed stage:

> The Reform shows the right direction for the country to take, though a difficult one to implement; and time has come for us to think about our future seriously ... I would like to note that integrating care and education under the responsibility of the education sector is the latest direction that is being adopted and considered by developed countries. But some years ago, their investment in early childhood, too, was justified as a means to increase the

female labour force and promote gender equality. Korea is in this earlier stage of development, but she will soon move into a more advanced stage. (UNESCO 2003, 2)

Up until this point, nobody, except a few ECE experts, had put the case in terms of social investment. The situation changed, however, after 2003. The policy context changed quite markedly as Korea's multiple socio-economic problems became increasingly evident. In reaction to the worsening economic conditions, the Roh government decided to recast the "productive welfare policy" paradigm it had inherited from its predecessor, the Kim Dae-jung government. Here two quite different streams of thinking merged: the neoliberal revisionist and the social capital advocate.

The neoliberal revisionist view – supported by policy bureaucrats from economic ministries such as the Ministry of Planning and Budget, the Ministry of Labour, and the Korea Development Institute – argued that Kim Dae-jung's productive welfare policy had been "inconsistent" and "old-fashioned" (Cho 2005, 84) and that the government should adopt a more "market-friendly productive welfare policy." There was also a growing understanding that Korea's economic problems were more than cyclical; rather, the root cause was postindustrial structural change. Their views echoed the advice tendered by international organizations such as the OECD, which was promoting governance and financial reforms. The group of Korean economic policy experts was thus informed by global discourse about postindustrial change and Third Way policies, particularly those being unrolled by the United Kingdom's New Labour. Economists such as Chae-Won Im, Jae-Jin Yang, Yong-Soon Kim, and Jae-Heung An argued that Korea needed to adopt a new social investment paradigm similar to that of the United Kingdom (W. Kim 2007). The economic bureaucrats thus focused on job creation, further expansion and refinement of the social safety net, more labour market flexibility, and increased support for human capital development through education and training (Cho 2005; Sul et al. 2006).

In contrast, the social capital perspective focused on the danger of social exclusion and disintegration resulting from growing economic polarization. Many researchers were dismayed by the decline in the level of civic participation and volunteer activities since the 1980s, seeing this as a sign of declining social trust and social cohesion (Joo, Lee, and Jo 2006). The "bipolarization" of the Korean economy was thought to contribute to the further deterioration of social cohesion. These researchers therefore called for government investment in social capital (e.g., social infrastructure work, support for NGOs, community development projects, and the building of communications and community facilities). Concern about the decline of social cohesion was not limited to sociologists and community groups: it also struck a chord with some economists. For instance, Choi (2009, 2), a senior fellow at the Korea Development Institute and a senior advisor for the Ministry of Budget and Finance, saw an economic rationale for ensuring social cohesion:

> A cohesive society is a society whose members have a shared value and a sense that they are engaged in a common enterprise, facing shared challenges, and that they belong to the same society. Hence social cohesion enables governments to better focus on growth vis-à-vis redistribution policies. This is why social cohesion is an important element in growth strategy in economics ... If a society has more equal income distribution, more people benefit from economic growth and will support policies that make economic growth happen – such as opening up the economy, investing in education, health, and R&D, investing in industries and social infrastructure, deregulating the economy etc.

Although different in their objectives, both perspectives converged with regard to the importance of social investment in the national development effort. Social welfare expansion, particularly ECEC and other forms of social care, made sense for both sets of actors. This strange by-product of the mixture of what Mahon (2006b) calls "inclusive liberalism" and social cohesion principles created an opening for economists and social welfare experts, enabling them to speak the same language when negotiating policy reforms. For those pursuing the ECE reform, this created a fortuitous moment in which to reframe and re-engage the social policy debate. Thus, despite the initial political setbacks, the process of policy learning and transfer continued as domestic policy actors worked to build their linkages with UNESCO and the OECD, in the process altering their understanding of ECEC and reframing it to fit Korean circumstances.

The Post-2003 Child-Care Reform Process: Advancing Social Care under the Social Investment Paradigm

The reform of Korea's child-care policies since 2003 provides an excellent case of a cross-sectoral policy-making process in which multiple actors converge around a single policy framework. Child-care reform addressed a number of important policy concerns represented in the interministerial group. First and foremost, it underscored the social investment paradigm's emphasis on human resource investment, with its futuristic orientation. In addition, the Ministry of Health and Welfare saw in child care an excellent way of addressing issues of fertility decline, population aging, obstacles to women's employment, and rising poverty. The Ministry of Gender Equality and Family saw in child care a way of achieving gender equality, while the Ministry of Labour and the Ministry of Planning and Budget saw in child care an economic stimulus due to the creation of a social-care market and, thus, the creation of much-needed jobs. Finally, MOEHRD and ECE policy experts saw child care as another chance to sort out the problems of parallel-track ECEC systems.

While all the members in the interministerial group agreed on the need to expand child care, they differed on the question of how to achieve this. The Ministry of Gender Equality and Family and its affiliated research institute, the Korean Women's Development Institute (KWDI), along with the Ministry of Health and Welfare, held numerous meetings on child-care strategy but failed to come up with a unified position on the system of delivery.

The Ministry of Gender Equality and Family supported the universal public child-care model favoured by the KWDI.[5] The KWDI's research had found significant public dissatisfaction with existing child-care policy. Most mothers surveyed felt that the child-care subsidies they received were too low and that there were not enough *public* child-care centres (the choice favoured by all mothers). The KWDI's understanding was also informed by the social democratic exemplars of Sweden and Denmark. Many of their researchers had studied the Scandinavian welfare state model and were convinced of the value of universal child care. They favoured the socialization of care, arguing that it would be more cost-effective for the government to provide public child-care services rather than to rely on subsidies.[6]

While the Ministry of Gender Equality and Family was supportive of universal public child care, the Ministry of Health and Welfare was divided. Many policy makers within the latter ministry saw the conversion to a public child-care system as impractical. Nearly 95 percent of child-care centres were private for-profit and not-for profit institutions, though almost all of them were regulated and partially funded through public money. Both ministries, however, agreed on the expansion of ECC as child care represented a significant portion of their policy portfolio. They also needed to respond to one of their biggest political constituencies – child care and child welfare service providers – who were feeling threatened by the MOEHRD's attempts to merge ECC with ECE.

MOEHRD was a cautious supporter of child-care expansion. The Presidential Commission on Education Reform's earlier failures to pass ECE reform law had taught ECE policy experts that it would be best to submit a new reform bill through MOEHRD rather than through a member's bill. ECE experts within MOEHRD had also learned from this experience that, initially, it was best to ensure the parallel expansion of ECE and child care and only later to pursue ECEC development through different channels.

Within the interministerial group, the biggest difference in ideas was between the economic ministries (the Ministry of Planning and Budget and the Ministry of Labour) and the social ministries (the Ministry of Gender Equality and Family and the Ministry of Health and Welfare). Moving beyond the issue of public versus private provision, the Ministry of Planning and Budget preferred the total deregulation of the child-care market, arguing that individual needs for child-care services can be most efficiently met by the market, while the Ministry of Labour saw in child-care expansion the potential for job creation in the private sector. While not entirely convinced of the merit of public provision, the Ministry of Health and Welfare was not comfortable with the Ministry of Planning and Budget's idea of total deregulation, being worried that quality might be sacrificed in the process. In contrast, the Ministry of Labour saw the burgeoning child-care market as an excellent opportunity to advance its interests in job creation and the facilitation of employment for women.

Outside of the interministerial group, the public debate on child-care policy reform also took place. Within the community, most NGOs and researchers supported the idea of publicly provided child-care services. With nearly 95 percent of the child-care providers in the private sector, the Private Childcare Providers' Association presented the largest opposition to the KWDI's universal public child-care proposal. Pointing to lack of efficiency and the need for flexibility in the public child-care system, the Private Childcare Providers' Association fiercely fought the expansion of public-sector child care. The Korean Childcare Teachers' Association (KCTA), the majority of whose membership worked in the private sector, was divided on the issue. Universal public child care presented both opportunities and constraints. Making child-care centres public would imply the formalization of employees' status as public service workers, bringing with it employment security, union representation, higher wages, and better working conditions. At the same time, it would also most likely entail stricter certification requirements, which might lead to retraining or decertifying many KCTA members. In the end, the KCTA accepted the private provision of child care.

Throughout 2005 and 2006, the interministerial committee debated the issue of child-care delivery. The committee's policy proposals were then given to the vice-ministers of all the relevant ministries, discussed within each ministry, and debated within the committee before an agreement was reached and presented to the president. The president then organized an all-ministers committee meeting and invited academic and policy experts in child care, ECE sectors, and members of civil society to discuss the plan. In 2005, the drop in the total fertility rate to 1.08, a historic low, gave the issue added salience.[7] Nevertheless, support for a universal public child-care proposal weakened in the face of other policy demands, such as job creation and fiscal control. At the same time, the Ministry of Health and Welfare had lost some of its earlier vested interest in child care when, in 2005, much of the family and child-care portfolio shifted over to the Ministry of Gender Equality and Family. Further, by this time, the Ministry of Health and Welfare's attention was focused on pension reform and long-term care insurance. The Ministry of Health and Welfare thus agreed to the Ministry of Planning and Budget's position to increase child-care subsidies rather than pushing for universal public child care. In the end, the reform resulted in a significant fiscal commitment to child care through subsidies to parents, while leaving the structure of private-sector-dominated provision.

Once the interministerial agreement had been reached, the programs unrolled rapidly. *Vision 2030* was followed by the government pledge to create 800,000 jobs through developing the social service sector. The Social Enterprise Promotion Law was introduced in 2007, formalizing state support for social enterprises and opening the door for business and NGO groups to apply for certification as a social enterprise (Korea Foundation for Working Together 2008). The Ministry of Labour had initiated a project to create social service jobs by providing grants to NGOs and had an annual budget of 7.3 billion won in 2003. With the introduction of the Social Enterprise Promotion Law, the project morphed into a multi-ministerial collaboration, with a total budget of 1.3 trillion won in 2007 (Ministry of Labour 2008). Much of the new social service job creations focused on child and elder care. From the Ministry of Labour's point of view, child-care reform was as much about stimulating the economy by seeding new social enterprises and creating new jobs as it was about ensuring care for children:

> Creating social service jobs has boosted our economy's growth potential as it has helped the not economically active population, including housewives and the aged, to be brought into the economically active population. In

particular, providing social services, such as child caring, housekeeping and patient caring, has liberated women from domestic work, which, in turn, has increased employment. The project to create social service jobs has not only created jobs for vulnerable groups of workers ... [but] has also played the role of providing social services which are in short supply, thereby largely contributing to supplying social services for low-income lower middle classes who want to get such services but have little purchasing power. The project has a great significance in that it has opened up new horizons by creating jobs in the social service sector, which is often called the third sector beyond the private and public sectors and needs to expand its share of employment through cooperation between NGOs and the government. (Ministry of Labour 2008)

In sum, child-care policy reform in Korea, which involved multiple-sector efforts to develop a child-care market, has led to the significant expansion of social care through financial subsidies to parents. The process leading to this was not a smooth one: it involved nearly two years of political debates, both inside and outside the government, in which multiple actors struggled to push forward their diverse policy agendas. In the end, pragmatic politics took over as actors, facing time pressures and fiscal constraints, made concessions. Nevertheless, it was largely because of the social investment paradigm that such expansionary social-care reform was possible in a time of fiscal constraint. Unlike social policy paradigms that so often pit economic development against social welfare, the social investment paradigm, with its promise of a possible win-win strategy, appealed to both sides. Child-care policy reform in Korea thus suggests a new kind of social policy thinking – a kind more rooted in political pragmatism than in ideological commitment.

Conclusion

This chapter examines the case of social-care expansion in Korea, focusing on changes in child-care and family-work harmonization policies since 2000. The recent expansion of social care in Korea reflects a combination of progressive and pragmatic approaches to social policy, both of which were informed by the social investment paradigm. In response to multiple socio-economic problems seen through the social investment lens, the Roh government viewed the expansion of social care as a strategy for simultaneously addressing diverse political demands: the creation of jobs, the provision of child-care and elder-care services, the better utilization of women's human capital, and the seeding of new engines of economic growth.

Social investment strategy is by no means unique to Korea; rather, the idea has been circulating within policy communities since the 1990s, and international policy experts have benefitted from the experiences of the Blair government's social investment experiments in the United Kingdom since 1997. Korean scholars and policy makers have been accumulating knowledge about social investment and testing it out with Kim Dae-jung's productive welfare policy since 1998. The Roh Moo-hyun administration, faced with a much greater imperative for policy innovation than was the Kim Dae-jung administration, went further and remodelled the latter's productive welfare policy. The new social investment strategy focused more directly on social care and targeted welfare expansion as a new economic growth engine.

The case of social-care expansion in Korea offers a few important lessons. First, it underscores the importance of the state's social policy not only in providing social welfare (as in the traditional notion of welfare state) but also in actively shaping the process and direction of economic development. Certainly, it can be argued that welfare state policies have always facilitated economic growth and industrial relations (e.g., through the provision of a social safety net and social insurance). Yet, their economic objectives have hitherto remained implicit. Simply put, traditionally, the principal role of the welfare state is to correct market failures, not to shape the market. The social investment paradigm differs from this in that it is explicitly market-focused and oriented towards economic growth. The social investment paradigm takes a more active role in shaping the market and thus directly affects modes of economic development. Korea may thus offer a new way of thinking about social policy and of conceptualizing the role of the welfare state.

Second, the Korean case adds to the emerging literature on social investment by demonstrating the different ways in which the social investment paradigm is being applied. Whereas social investment policies in the United Kingdom were primarily aimed at mobilizing a growing number of unemployed youth, women, and industrial workers who were dependent on income assistance, Korea's social investment policies were more focused on creating jobs in the service sector and on mobilizing women's human capital in response to population aging. British social investment thus focused more on skills development and adult retraining through education. In the case of Korea, much social investment focused on the expansion of social care for two population groups – children and the elderly – and the cumulative outcome was the commodification of women's unpaid care work. In both the United Kingdom and Korea, social investment policies contained a significant gender dimension, but they differed in gender specificity as their targets differed from one another. The Korean case thus illustrates how a global social policy can result in different applications in different contexts.

Finally, the Korean case also highlights the current intensity and importance of global policy learning and transfer. Over the last few decades, increased economic globalization has led to increased attempts by regional and global institutions to harmonize social and economic policies. As we have seen in this chapter, in Korea, the pressure for global policy learning and transfer do not simply come from the bottom in the form of domestic demand for policy innovations. It also comes from the top in the form of a global movement towards policy harmonization. Policy recommendations from international organizations such as the OECD and the IMF thus serve as important tools of global policy coordination. To be sure, there is a genuine national interest in adopting and conforming to international policy culture. For recently developed countries (like Korea), the degree of their social policy alignment with that of exemplar nations is an important measure of their social development, which, by providing them with international recognition, feeds their sense of national prestige. In sum, the directions and the motivations for global policy learning and transfer are far more complex and multidirectional now than they were before. The Korean case thus cautions us to approach policy learning and transfers from a multidimensional perspective.

6

Reimagined Intimate Relations
Elder and Child Care in Japan since the 1990s

YUKI TSUJI

Elder- and child-care policies in Japan have changed dramatically over the last decade. In contrast to other OECD countries, where neoliberal restructuring or the retrenchment of welfare states has facilitated the privatization of care, Japan, like Korea (see Peng, this volume), has promoted the socialization of elder and child care to address the problems of an aging population and a rapidly declining birthrate. While an expansion of social care is expected to transform the gendered division of care for the elderly and children, the redistribution of care within society may give rise to new differentiations among people who provide and need care, depending on their social positions as constituted by gender, race, class, sexuality, age, and nationality. This chapter, which traces the policy-making processes of Japanese elder- and child-care policy reforms, analyzes the political debates surrounding the introduction and revision of public LTCI for the elderly and policies for countering the declining birthrate. It attempts to answer the following questions: (1) In what ways have competing discourses and ideas affected and shaped the socialization of care in Japan since the 1990s? (2) How have the domestic discussions on social care been influenced by the international discourses of care? and (3) How have identities, subjectivities, and relations between people been transformed by the reorganization of social care?

This chapter investigates the ways in which the socialization of care has been influenced by three types of political discourse: neoliberalism, gender equality, and familialism. First, it examines the debate on the form of care provision (i.e., the issue of cash versus services), revealing both collaboration and contention among these discourses. Second, it examines the intersections between domestic and international discourses of care, with particular reference to the OECD's *Babies and Bosses* project, which looks at Japanese work/care balance policy. The key argument, however, is that the resulting redistribution of care has been accompanied by the reimagining of intimate relations, especially family relations. While care for the elderly has been labelled a "burden" for family caregivers, young parents are still expected to take all responsibility for raising their children by providing not only a good (expensive) education but also love, affection, and care.

The Literature on Care and an Analytical Framework
Feminist scholars have elaborated the concept of care as a challenge to existing intellectual frameworks in various disciplines. Feminist political economists have pointed out that care work (or "social reproduction") carried out by women (and racialized men) is necessary to maintain the capitalist economy. They have demonstrated that organizations of production and social reproduction in the capitalist political economy are constituted by social hierarchy based on gender, race, and class relations (Barker 2005). In describing the different ways care is organized, feminists have made a substantial contribution to the study of welfare regimes. Thus Daly and Lewis (2000) introduce the concept of social care as a basis for comparing the development and transformation of welfare regimes. In various ways, welfare states distribute three dimension of care (i.e., cost, labour, and responsibility) between sectors (i.e., state, market, family, and community) and between people divided by gender, race, and class. On this basis, Daly and Lewis distinguish European welfare states according to the degree and nature of collectivization and privatization of care (288-89).

Scholars informed by the ethics-of-care approach challenge the perception of autonomous, independent subjects assumed in Western liberal thought. Liberal thought assumes that only autonomous and independent citizens participate in the public sphere, where they discuss public matters. This perception of citizens excludes those who need and provide care (i.e. women, children, ill/disabled, and the elderly). To counter this, feminist scholars insist that no person can survive without care and that human beings are fundamentally interdependent. This battle over the conceptualization of subjects in relation to care is, as Tronto (1993 and this volume) argues, political because caring activities produce power relations between people. Not only can those who are most powerful in a society ignore the needs of care altogether, but there are differences in social statuses between those who engage in different phases of care: "caring about, and taking care of, are the duties of the powerful. Caregiving and care-receiving are left to the less powerful" (Tronto 1993, 114). This distinction between phases of caring can be considered the distinction between care as the labour (caregiving and care-receiving) and care as cost and responsibility (caring about, taking care of). The kind of caring in which a person is involved not only suggests his/her social position but also constitutes his/her subjectivity. Those who neither need nor provide care can imagine themselves as rational, independent, and autonomous subjects. At the same time, the normalization of an independent, autonomous subject leads to the marginalization of those subjectivities who recognize the interdependence between human beings. Hierarchical relations between subjects involve gender, race, and class relations. "Care," then, is a concept that yields simultaneous insight into the processes of social organization, subject formation, and power relations.

Expansion of social care affects, and is affected by, changes in the modern family, a unit based on intimate relations between members who share resources and spaces, and who maintain mutual emotional engagements (Levy 2005). Political actors who try to change the social organization of care must take into account people's expectations and actual intimate relations and families. At the same time, the reorganization of social care is accompanied by a shift of boundaries between the private and the public spheres, and the reimagination of family and intimate relations. To some extent, the expansion of public responsibility for care disrupts the conceptual and practical link between care, the private, family, and intimacy. The rise of social concern about care has, in turn, the potential to transform the perception of the public, which has been thought of as being composed of independent and autonomous citizens.

Care thus has multiple dimensions, which are socially constructed and contingent upon time and place. What, then, facilitates the reorganization of these multiple dimensions of care? While structural change can contribute to the reorganization of care, such changes are given meaning through discourse and discursive contests. As Schmidt (2003) argues, political actors employ discourses to construct and legitimize their policy programs, and such discourses contain both cognitive (based on empirical reasoning) and normative (appealing to socially shared values) arguments. Discourses for policy changes provide people with alternative explanations of society and different perceptions of interests from those provided in the existing welfare state. Discourses regarding social-care policy reforms are implicitly or explicitly based on the perception of particular subjects who need and deliver care, proper sites for caring, and relations between people who engage in care. These discourses not only affect policy changes but also reflect the transformation of social structure and human relations, such as changes in family composition and gender relations. With regard to elder- and childcare policy reforms in Japan, three types of political discourse – gender equality, neoliberalism, and familialism – have influenced the reorganization of social care.

Neoliberalism has emerged as a repudiation of the Keynesian welfare state in attempting not only to reduce government's control over the market economy but also to introduce market rationality into the management of public policies. As Brown suggests (2005, 40), neoliberalism is a constructivist project that "produces rational actors and imposes a market rationale for decision making" in all domains of society. Citizens are required to be entrepreneurs as well as consumers in all aspects of their lives, and social policies are redesigned to provide incentives to transform citizens into such neoliberal subjects. In terms of care and social reproductive work, neoliberalism tends to ignore the way these activities contribute to the maintenance and reproduction of the capitalist economy. Policies following a neoliberal logic, therefore, can lead to the decline of social reproduction.

The goal of gender equality includes not only providing equal opportunities for women and men but also recognizing differences between as well as within men and women and, moreover, transforming social structures and power relationships through which dominance and subordination between men and women are reproduced. Gender mainstreaming comprises the political and administrative practices of integrating the perspective of gender equality into all areas of policy-making processes and assessments that have been adopted by many international organizations, development agencies, and national governments (True 2003). It aims not only at incorporating "women" and their perspectives into decision making but also at transforming frameworks of existing social and institutional settings that have been based on privileged male perspectives. When introduced and practised in different national contexts, however, the contents of gender equality in gender mainstreaming policies have been variously interpreted (Verloo 2005, 354-57). Feminist scholars agree that gender mainstreaming may promote the equal participation of women and men in the labour force and facilitate the political representation of women. At the same time, by employing the discourse of neoliberalism (favouring "productive" activities in the market economy and devaluing social reproductive work), it could generate new hierarchal relationships between subjects differently situated in class and race relations.

Following Leitner (2003), familialism may be defined as an ideology that asserts that care should be primarily provided by family members. Familial policies guarantee family caregivers "(1) time rights (such as parental leave and care leave), (2) direct and indirect transfers for caring (such as cash benefits and tax reductions) and (3) social rights attached to caregiving like individual pension rights or the (partial) inclusion in other social security schemes or derived rights for non-employed wives (husbands)" (Leitner 2003, 358). In contrast, defamilializing policies "aim at unburdening the family in its caring function, like the public provision of child care and/or social services or the (public subsidy of) care provision through the market" (ibid.). In principle, familialism does not have any preference as to the gender of family caregivers. Feminists might be able to employ a familialist discourse to promote male engagement in child care in the family. In some cases, familialism plays a supplemental role to neoliberalism by promoting the privatization of care; in other cases, it might blame neoliberalism for the breakdown of the "traditional" form of the family and require the state to adopt policies for protecting it.

The relationship between these three political discourses depends on the social context and the balance among social forces. It is therefore necessary to look at the national context in which political discourses operate and social realities are framed. At the same time, it is important to be aware that these three discourses do not operate exclusively within national boundaries. Along with the development of globalization and the emergence of supranational institutions for global governance, national politics has become more open to the influence of international political discourses, as pointed out by Mahon (2006a; this volume), while international discourses themselves are sometimes constructed by the leadership of national governments and other agencies (such as NGOs). In addition, as both Robinson (this volume) and Onuki (this volume) argue, nations are located in and constitutive of the global political economy. Thus, national analyses of, and solutions to, social problems can reflect a process of transnational policy learning (Peng, this volume).

Examination of the debate on forms of socializing care – cash benefits versus service provision – can yield insight into the intersection of these three discourses and reveal shifts in power relations. The issue of cash or services involves the decision on how to share the cost and labour of care (Daly and Lewis 2000). It is important to grasp the organization of the cash and service dimensions of the welfare state. While cash benefits facilitate family care, the institutionalization of public child care and/or the commercialization of child care promote the defamilialization of child care and facilitate women's participation in the labour force (Leitner 2003). In sum, the issue of cash or services is critical in determining the ways in which the state and society regulate care provisioning and connect or separate family and care (Jenson 1997).

I focus my analysis of the Japanese debate on how this complicated issue is framed by political actors when discussing social-care policies. Although, in principle, the three political discourses can position themselves in various ways on the issue of cash or services, there seems to be a general tendency. First, from the perspective of gender equality, providing care services is seen as important for achieving economic equality as it makes it possible for women to remain in the paid labour force. In contrast, familialism favours cash provision in order to facilitate family caregiving, while neoliberalism prefers private care arrangements (i.e., care delivered either through the market or by the family rather than through either public care provision or cash benefits to family caregivers).

Elder- and Child-Care Policy Reforms in Japan since the 1990s

Japanese social policies began to undergo dramatic changes in the 1990s, from the social assistance system *(sochi seido)*, whereby a minority of people without income and family support were recognized as recipients of welfare by the state, to the contractual system, whereby a broad range of citizens became providers as well as consumers of social services. As Peng (2002, 412) notes, "the 1990s was an important decade of social care expansion in Japan." The LTCI scheme, which aims to "shift care provisions for the elderly from a means-tested public welfare program to one based on the principle of social right" (401), was enacted in 1997 and implemented in 2000. Paid parental leave started in 1995, and the number and variety of child-care facilities and services have been increased by the state's initiatives, known as the "Angel Plan" and the "New Angel Plan." These changes have been facilitated by demographic changes, the transformation of gender relations, and the opening of the political opportunity structure towards new actors during Japan's political realignment (Boling 1998, 2003; Eto 2001a, 2001b; Peng 2002, 2004).

It would, however, be too simple to see these policy reforms as a coherent, unidirectional process. The changes have been contentious, giving rise to important fractures. In designing new measures and policies, diverse actors have tried to incorporate contradictory ideas and values regarding gender, family, and the market economy. After years of Liberal Democratic rule, in the 1990s, Japanese politics experienced successive coalition governments. The long-governing Liberal Democratic Party was thus forced to accept demands from centre-left parties for certain progressive programs, including gender mainstreaming, which was institutionalized in 1999.[1] The socialization of elder care was promoted during this period. Since 2001, Prime Minister Jun'ichirō Koizumi has promoted the neoliberal restructuring of the state and society, while at the same time showing his support for the realization of gender equality by appointing female cabinet ministers. At the same time, Koizumi's reforms faced opposition from conservatives opposing gender equality and "established interest groups" resisting the neoliberal restructuring of the state and society. In what follows I look at (1) the introduction (and revision) of public LTCI and (2) the socialization of child care. The issue of cash versus service provision arose in both debates.

Long-Term Care Insurance

In the traditional Japanese-style patriarchal system *(ie seido)*, it was taken for granted that a daughter-in-law (the oldest son's wife) cared for the frail elder parents-in-law (Long and Harris 2000, 30). Since the late 1980s, however, Japanese society has had to listen to the concerns of families who have found it increasingly difficult to provide such intrafamilial care. The idea of public LTCI was proposed in December 1994 by the Ministry of Health and Welfare (which merged with the Ministry of Labour in 2001 and was renamed the Ministry of Health, Labour and Welfare [MHLW]), opening up a debate about whether and how to establish LTCI in Japan. Advocates of LTCI widely disseminated the slogan "socialization of care," meaning that society would share the labour and cost of elder care (Tsutsui and Muramatsu 2005, 522). The bill was passed in 1997 and was finally implemented in 2000.

The main lines of the LTCI system can be summarized as follows: (1) expansion of the coverage of beneficiaries and public care services, (2) change of the financial resources, and (3) participation of new care providers. First, LTCI expanded potential care beneficiaries from low-income seniors lacking family support to the overall population aged sixty-five years old and above, and it increased the quantity and variety of public care services (such as visiting nurses, day care, short-stay services, and housekeeping services). Second, in terms of financial resources, while the previous social security system for the elderly was funded entirely by the government, the LTCI system is financed half by social insurance contributions from people aged forty and older and half by government revenues. In addition, users pay 10 percent of the cost of care services provided by LTCI.[2] Finally, the introduction of LTCI facilitated the entry of private businesses into the care market by relaxing state regulation, though, in fact, prices, wages, contents, and quality of care services are still regulated by the central and local governments.

From the beginning of the 1990s, the Ministry of Health and Welfare took the initiative regarding the introduction of the LTCI system, but it was not the only actor. The Liberal Democratic Party coalition government provided access to the policy-making process for citizens groups and the Japanese Trade Union Confederation (RENGO), which were demanding the socialization of care through the introduction of the public care insurance system. Women's groups played a particularly important role here (Eto 2001a, 2001b). In contrast, business representatives, such as the Japan Federation of Employers' Association (NIKKEIREN), argued against the social insurance system, claiming that employers could not afford their share of the contribution. In addition, the representatives of local governments worried about the growth of their fiscal and administrative burdens as local governments were expected to run the LCTI system on a daily basis. Nevertheless, since public opinion was clearly in favour of the introduction of a new system, the MHW focused its attention on how to introduce the universal elder-care system through the social insurance principle.

Shortly after the introduction of LTCI, however, the Japanese government began to contemplate its revision in order to constrain the growth of government expenditure. The reforms to the LTCI Law in 2005 introduced the concept of a "preventive approach to care" *(kaigo yobō)*, which was aimed at preventing (or at least delaying) the aggravation of symptoms of aging (MHLW 2004). Options such as strength training and nutrition improvement were incorporated into the LTCI menu.

The effects of the new LTCI system are divided by gender and class. The introduction of LTCI changed the concept of public care from the stigmatized residual assistance for low-income elderly to a universal right. At the same time, some, due to low and unstable incomes, cannot pay the insurance premiums – an ever more frequent phenomenon as irregular employment is now being experienced by male workers. The 10 percent payment for care services also puts pressure on budgets in low-income households. In sum, LTCI provides a benefit to the middle- and upper classes but not to the lower class (Tsutsui and Muramatsu 2005, 525). Considering the income and age gaps between elderly men and women, this issue is more serious for the latter than it is for the former. Older women are often without finances as well as without physical help from their spouses.

Another controversial issue in the LTCI debate was whether to provide a cash allowance to family caregivers. Some conservative politicians, especially those representing rural communities, supported the introduction of cash allowance to family caregivers, claiming that family members' caring for the elderly is a good Japanese tradition. Feminist scholars and activists strongly opposed this, arguing that cash provisions would simply consolidate the gendered division of care labour. Keiko Higuchi, a feminist who was a member of the Advisory Council on Elders' Health and Welfare as well as the chair of the Women's Association for Improving an Aging Society, opposed a cash allowance, arguing that paying money would slow down the institutionalization of the public care services in communities and that family care without social intervention might impair the quality of care. Moreover, as a cash payment would facilitate the concentration of care labour on a particular member of the family, typically a woman, such a move would contradict the goal of gender equality (Higuchi 1999).

At the same time, since paying family caregivers can be interpreted as recognizing the value of unpaid care labour, it could reward (emotionally and financially) women who have already engaged in family care for a long time (Keefe and Rajnovich 2007). Thus, some favoured financial support for families (Kikuchi 2010), which is understandable as family caregivers found it hard to secure jobs after their long absence from the labour market. Yet, unless care labour is recognized as "real" work, cash benefits will be smaller than wages in the labour market, which, in turn, adversely affects the working conditions of care workers outside the family.[3] In the end, a cash allowance was incorporated into LTCI but only under strict conditions, according to which family caregivers with home care worker certificates *(kaigo herupa)* could be paid when they provided home-care services to family members (although the amount of time spent on families should not exceed half of the caregiver's total work time). Otherwise, family caregivers in low-income households could receive 100,000 yen per year when they did not use LTCI services.

Finally, it is worth noting that the rise of social and political concern about elder care in Japan had an impact on the construction of international discourse, especially within the OECD. Thus, at the 1996 OECD Summit in Lyon, Japanese prime minister Ryūtarō Hashimoto argued for the "Initiative for a Caring World," proposing that each country share its knowledge and experience of social security policies with other countries in order to deal with an aging society and to build a better society for the next generation. The OECD subsequently used the term "caring world" as the title of the report in which it set out new directions for social policy reform. Thus, care became a public issue at the international level as well as at the national level.

The Socialization of Child Care or Measures to Increase the Birthrates?

When Japan's fertility rate plunged to 1.57 in 1989, the issue of the declining birthrate hit the political agenda. In the first phase of child-care policy reforms, however, the falling birthrate was considered a temporary phenomenon resulting from the tendency of women to marry later (MHW 1991; Cabinet Office 2004). At this point, the debate on the declining birthrate focused on measures to encourage women to have children. Paid parental leave was legislated and implemented in 1995, and the Angel Plan was enacted in 1994, with the aim of increasing the number and variety of child-care services, including nursery schools and after-school care for children. Nevertheless, the child-care norm remained unchanged: child care should be delivered primarily within family, and the role of the state and society should be limited to providing supplementary support for family-based child care (Cabinet Office 2004). The persistence of the ideal of family-based child care was evident when the income replacement rate for paid parental leave was settled at only 25 percent of the parent's salary. This made it difficult for a primary earner in a family (usually the father) to take one-year parental leave. The replacement rate was increased to 40 percent in 2001, but it is still low considering the rather large gender pay gap in Japan (32.0 percent) when compared with the OECD average (18.5 percent) (OECD 2007).

In contrast to the first round of reforms, since 1998, measures for increasing the birthrate have been explicitly linked to the promotion of gender equality. The 1998 *Annual Report on Health and Welfare* required fathers' participation in child rearing, arguing that promoting gender equality would encourage people to have children (MHW 1998). In addition to the government, business circles and trade unions accepted the concept of gender equality. The Japan Association of Corporate Executives, the Japan Federation of Employers' Association, and the Tokyo Chamber of Commerce and Industry issued statements proclaiming their efforts to introduce measures to increase the birthrate. In 1999, NIKKEIREN cooperated with the Japanese Trade Union Confederation (RENGO) to construct a joint declaration on their commitment to taking measures against the declining birthrate. The joint declaration admits that it is necessary to "alleviate burdens of women in terms of childbirth, child rearing, and housekeeping and to have men share domestic responsibility." It also promises that both labour and management would try to promote the employment of women with children, introduce flexible working hours and teleworking, and reduce working hours (NIKKEIREN and RENGO 2000).[4] Prime Minister Koizumi also promised to expand public support for child raising, while the state minister in charge of economic and fiscal policy, Heizō Takenaka, insisted that a structural reform of the working environment was necessary because the existing norms and institutions, based on the male breadwinner model, had produced such problems as long working hours and discrimination against women and the elderly (Cabinet Office 2002a; Takeda 2008).

International discourses have helped to encourage the introduction of work/care balance policies. Thus, the OECD's *Babies and Bosses* assessment of Japanese policies was delivered at the Committee of Equal Employment in the Labour Policy Council in the MHLW. It contained proposals for work/care balance policies such as expanding paid care leaves and the introduction of short-time regular employment (MHLW 2003b). In the discussions in the Diet, the positive relationship between female labour force participation and fertility rate, highlighted in the OECD report, was sometimes employed to legitimize work/care balance policies (National Diet Library 2006). The CEDAW report was referred to by a labour representative in the Committee of Equal Employment, in calling for the promotion of work/care balance for *male* workers (MHLW 2003a). Although the reports and recommendations by international organizations do not have the power to force the Japanese government to follow their advice, they do offer policy options on which domestic political actors may draw in constructing their policy proposals. In addition, the statistical data based on scientific research methods in these reports provided material that enabled domestic actors to justify their political claims.

Expansion of public support for child raising has been influenced not only by gender equality but also by neoliberal discourse. While the phrase "socialization of child raising" has appeared in the mass media, the more frequent phrase is "investment in the future" (Cabinet Office 2008a). The socialization of child care has, in fact, facilitated the deregulation of the child-care market, and it has also promoted the delegation of child-care planning to local governments, in accordance with the decentralization of the Japanese political system.[5] In this respect, the "third way approach" towards child care presented in *Babies and Bosses* (Mahon 2006a) seems to be shared by Japanese child-care policies. Thus, while gender equality's alliance with the neoliberal agenda has given it added legitimacy and has helped to bring about the expansion of public support for working women with children, at the same time, it poses the risk of subordinating gender equality to the logic of neoliberalism, as exemplified by the destabilization of employment in every sector.

As in long-term care insurance, the issue of cash or service provision has been important in the child-care debates. The issue was discussed in meetings of the Advisory Panel on the Promotion of Measures for Reversing the Declining Birthrate, held from November 2005 to May 2006. The panel, composed of experts in gender, employment, family relations, and child care, and chaired by Kuniko Inoguchi (the minister in charge of dealing with the declining birthrate), repeatedly emphasized the need to reduce working hours, adopt work/care balance policies, and expand child-care services before increasing economic assistance to families. Without these structural changes in the labour market, workplaces, and communities, it reasoned, cash benefits to families with children might reinforce the existing division of labour, according to which only women take care of children (Cabinet Office 2006a).

Nevertheless, there was strong support for cash benefits for child care among politicians. Only three days after the release of the Advisory Panel's final report, Inoguchi submitted *Proposal on New Measures for Increasing the Birthrate* to the Council of Fiscal and Economic Policy. This proposal included financial support measures such as the provision of cost-free childbirth, cash benefits to children under three years old, and tax reduction (Cabinet Office 2006b). The Advisory Panel experts protested, arguing that the proposal ignored its advice. Inoguchi insisted that the proposal sought to satisfy citizens' demands for financial support while also recognizing the importance of a changing working environment and the need for care services. Since the Advisory Panel lacked political and institutional power, its focus on gender equality was easily pushed aside by vote-seeking political actors, who sought to increase financial support for families. In April 2007, the child allowance for children under three years old was raised to 10,000 yen per month, and again, in the 2009 Lower House general election, the Democratic Party proposed increasing child allowance to 26,000 yen per month for children under fifteen years of age. It also promised to reduce the costs of secondary education. Although there were arguments for and against these proposals, the Democratic Party successfully attracted the attention of voters, especially among the young generation.

Reimagined Intimate Relations

The socialization of elder care and child care has been accompanied by the reimagination of intimate family relations. To sum up, while elder care has been recognized as a burden for family members, child raising is still expected to be an enjoyable experience for parents. Family responsibility for elder care has accordingly decreased since the 1980s, as is reflected in the political agreement to socialize elder care (MHW 1998). The introduction of the LTCI system, in turn, justified the transformation of social values regarding familial elder care obligations. More and more, the Japanese have come to think that children (and daughters-in-law) do not necessarily have to take care of their elderly parents (Cabinet Office 2003). This does not mean that the elderly are detached from their children, only that people do not want to place a heavy burden on their sons and daughters. Elderly parents seem to be expected to take care of themselves, supplemented by social-care services. In other words, the concept of "self-responsibility" has been introduced to the subjectivities of elderly people. In contrast, young parents' responsibility for their children's education and welfare has not been lightened, even though public support has expanded. As Honda (2008) points out, the importance of "home education" *(katei kyōiku)* is increasingly emphasized in the mass media and political discourses. While, to a certain degree, the Japanese government institutionalized early childhood education, the term "home education" suggests the familialization of childhood education. Today's parents are enjoined to provide not only a good education but also love and care so that their children can develop a wide range of abilities (e.g., communication skills) that will be useful in a postindustrial society. In fact, it is mothers who are primarily responsible for home education. Without help from husbands, who often work until late at night, mothers who spend all day with their babies sometimes experience emotional breakdowns or even abuse their children.[6] Under such circumstances, women seem to prefer to opt out of marriage and child rearing altogether (Schoppa 2006a, 2006b).

The shift of public concern from elder care to child care and the reimagination of intimate relations between parents and children illustrate the normalization of the neoliberal family and neoliberal subjectivity in Japanese society. Children, who are the future labour force, are indispensable resources for a nation that hopes to maintain a successful capitalist economy. The state seems to be trying to construct citizens who "naturally" desire to have a family and children, and this shows the subtle alliance between neoliberalism and familialism.[7] Both the state and the business sector propose building a society in which people hope to have children, but they do so without challenging the neoliberal organization of society. The neoliberal family and neoliberal subjectivity marginalize certain people (especially men), placing them in the lower strata of the "marriage market" if they cannot afford the expenses of child raising. Neoliberal society is also gendered and racialized in so far as women from other Asian countries are invited to Japan as care workers for the elderly but not as citizens (Onuki, this volume). In the elder-care market, the average wage of care workers remains low, and the state has recreated the gendered difference between professional caregivers and home helpers. There is no sign that the public will be reconceptualized according to an ethics of care.

Conclusion

This chapter tries to link national and domestic forms of social reorganization by investigating the relationship between social care policy reforms and the transformation of parent-child relations. It argues that three types of political discourse – neoliberalism, gender equality, and familialism – have influenced the perceptions of problems relating to an aging population and a diminishing number of children, and have shaped the processes involved in reforming social care in Japan. Through these processes, intimate relations, especially family relations, have been reimagined, and this, in turn, affects the development of social-care policies. Although the socialization of elder care and child care transformed, to a certain extent, the boundary of public responsibility for care, it could end up redrawing the boundary of the family, including young parents and children while excluding elderly parents. Reforms in elder-care and child-care policies have not been completed, nor are their implications regarding the transformation of gender relations clear.[8] New social, economic, and political environments will lead to a reorganization of how care for the elderly and children is delivered, and this, as ever, will involve gender, class, and race.

PART 3

The Transnational Ethics of Care

7

Care Ethics and the Transnationalization of Care
Reflections on Autonomy, Hegemonic Masculinities, and Globalization

FIONA ROBINSON

> *A global demand exists for labour whose core component consists of "women's work." By this I mean sex, childcare and housework. Demand exceeds supply of female citizens of affluent states willing to provide these services in the market. By and large, this has not led to a decline in the demand for commercial sex, a systemic redistribution of unpaid domestic labour between the sexes, or an increased market valorization of "women's work." Instead, migrant women from poor countries are recruited to top up the deficit at low cost.*
>
> – Audrey Macklin (2003, 454)

This chapter asks what kind of moral perspective is required in order to make sense of the ethical dilemmas that arise in a situation in which millions of women from income-poor, peripheral states migrate to more affluent countries to do the work that is "associated with a wife's traditional role – child care, homemaking and sex" (Ehrenreich and Hochschild 2002, 4). This situation is usually causally linked to social and demographic transformations in the nature, extent, and location of paid work, notably the increase in women's labour force participation. Recent estimates show women as the sole, primary, or coequal earners in more than half of American families (3). In Canada, between 1960 and 2000, women's share of the labour force increased from 25 to 48 percent (Heymann, Earle, and Hanchate 2004). In the absence of accessible, affordable, universal child-care programs in income-rich countries, many women working outside the home now purchase transnationally the reproductive labour that they no longer have time to provide.

The transnational demand for care providers (usually women) is reflected in migration flows. Between 1985 and 1990, the number of women migrating to another country increased at a faster rate than the number of men (United Nations Development Fund for Women 2000, 31). By the beginning of the twenty-first century, women comprised almost 50 percent of the world's 120 million migrants, many of them seeking reproductive work in the nearest comparatively rich country (Agathangelou 2004, 5). In countries like the Philippines, Indonesia, and Sri Lanka, female migrant workers significantly outstrip male migrant workers (UNIFEM 2005). While the focus of this migration tends to be on nannies and domestic workers, the migration of women for sex work is a substantial part of this trend. As Agathangelou (2004, 6) points out, "desire industries" constitute one of the fastest-growing employment sectors for working-class migrant women.

This chapter asks why this simple "supply-and-demand" equation is usually seen as an adequate explanation of the globalization of women's domestic labour and sex work, and why normative considerations are often removed from view. To help find the answer to these questions, I employ a critical feminist ethics of care as an ontological and normative lens. Care ethics starts from the position that all people exist in webs of relations with others, relying on those others for their care and, hence, their security. While there are many versions of care ethics, I defend a critical, feminist version of the ethics of care, which eschews the epistemological certainty of moral foundationalism. In other words, it does not valorize caring relations or caring values as either intrinsically morally superior or more desirable based on their "femininity." On the contrary, as a critical ethics, it is committed to understanding how power works *through* ethics. Thus, it asks how particular moral discourses, and the behaviour and institutions they license, may lead to the exclusion or suffering of particular groups of people. This approach to ethics does not mean that it is never possible to say which values and moral principles are better or worse than others. Yet, it does insist that there can never be values or principles that are always, for everyone, morally right; rather, it locates those values and practices in specific temporal, spatial, and social contexts and seeks to uncover who gains, and who loses, in these contexts.

In the context of transnational care work, this approach focuses on the mutually constitutive nature of the global political economy of gender and race, the normative structures of hegemonic masculinities, and the moral discourses of "womanhood," "family," "exoticism," and "national security." An ethics of care that is both critical and feminist can help to uncover and elucidate the moral discourses and normative structures that govern the global distribution of "intimate services" as well as the responsibility and demand for those services. Moreover, as a feminist ethics, it can assist in revealing the reasons that women, especially racialized women, are responsible for sex work, as they are for "housework" and "care work," and why there is relatively little critical moral reflection on this in the context of relations of gender and race at the global level. Thus, this chapter asks why women – particularly "exotic," racialized women – are regarded as the natural providers of caring and "intimate" labour. How do the politics of race and gender work with discourses and structures of neoliberal globalization to ensure that the moral questions raised by these issues remain shielded from view and, thus, from critical scrutiny? What is the relationship between the "glitzy" world of deregulated global finance, produce, and trade – often referred to simply as "globalization," the policies and practices of states (including peripheral states) – and the transnational regime of sexualized, racialized "labour intimacy"? (Chang and Ling 2000, 27). Why is it that increasing demand for care work in affluent, income-rich countries has not increased the value of that labour? What kinds of normative structures are in place to ensure that care work retains its universally low status – both in terms of its market and societal value? Finally, how have the "moralizing" discourses of sex, criminality, and security obscured the gendered and raced political economy of globalized sex work?

In an effort to address these questions, the first part of this chapter sets out the characteristics of a critical, feminist ethics of care, focusing particularly on distinguishing this approach to ethics from traditional rights-based, universalist, and impartialist views of ethics. It also, however, seeks to explain why care ethics must be both feminist and critical if it is to provide a normative framework that is ultimately transformative of existing, oppressive relations of gender and race in the global political economy.

The second part of the chapter explores the relationship between the transnationalization of women's domestic labour and the moral discourses surrounding "care." In so doing, it seeks to elucidate the relationship between the empirical observation that women do most of the world's care work and the normative structures supporting the feminization and racialization of this work. In most societies, this feminization is largely taken for granted as it reflects traditional gendered divisions of labour; it is supported ideologically in both developed and industrialized economies (and by many international organizations and financial institutions) as well as by most religions and cultures (Kurian 2006, 157-58). The important role of hegemonic norms of masculinity, however, in legitimizing and sustaining the feminization of care work, is rarely examined. This section explores the discourses of hegemonic masculinity at a variety of different levels in order to uncover the role they play in supporting the transnationalization of women's labour. It also seeks to demonstrate how the contemporary transnationalization of domestic, care, and sex work is a feature of dual processes of globalization that are racially and spatially constituted. Gender hierarchies and constructions of gender cannot shed light on the moral dimensions of these questions unless gender is seen as intersecting race, class, and geo-political hierarchies.

The third part of the chapter introduces the particular challenges surrounding the moral discourses of sex work and attempts to uncover the normative links between sex work and more traditional forms of "care work." Although the "moralizing" discourses surrounding sexuality, criminality, and national security have meant that sex work is regarded as fundamentally different from other kinds of social reproductive labour, the lens of care can also illuminate the ethics and politics of transnational sex work.

The Ethics of Care and Women's Work

> *The domestic and caring sector is often referred to as feudal, involving servitude and servility. How is it that these social phenomena are looked on so uncritically within Western societies?*
>
> – Laura Agustin (2003, 387)

While the earliest conceptualizations of the ethics of care were constructed around empirical data used to build hypotheses in moral psychology, a number of more recent feminist accounts of care ethics have been self-consciously political. Indeed, it may be more correct to say that many feminist scholars took seriously the powerful political implications of Carol Gilligan's (1982) early findings regarding the gendered differences in responses to a variety of moral dilemmas. While a few feminist scholars were wary – of essentialism, of the reification of stereotypes, or of Western bias – a large group of feminists from a variety of disciplines have recognized the enormous significance of bringing "care," as both a set of values and a type of work, out of the "private" sphere. In so doing, these feminists are seeking not to "transfer" care from one sphere to another (i.e., the public sphere) but, rather, to deconstruct the gendered dichotomies that have created two separate realms of human existence.

While accounts of the nature of the ethics of care differ, it is possible to isolate a number of key attributes of the substance of care ethics that distinguish it from other approaches to ethics. Joan Tronto's well-known formulation of care ethics highlights the importance in this approach to ethics not of moral values or principles as such but, rather, of *practices* as constitutive of morality. These include attentiveness, responsibility, nurturance, compassion, and meeting others' needs (Tronto 1993, 3). Building on these central moral practices, I argue that a critical feminist ethics of care must include reference to not only the substance of morality but also to key ontological and methodological assumptions that provide the groundwork for thinking about morality in this way. Thus, an ethics of care includes the following: a relational ontology, which conceptualizes selves as fully relational – existing in and through complex, constitutive webs or relations with others; a focus on attention, responsiveness, and responsibility to the needs of particular others as core substantive moral values; a commitment to addressing moral problems in the historical and spatial contexts of real, lived experiences; and, finally, a reconceptualization of traditional understandings of the nature of and relationship between the "public" and the "private" spheres.

Relational ontology could be described as the core of this approach to ethics. Care ethicists argue that the dominant moral and political ontology of autonomy – of isolated, self-reliant moral selves – does not adequately reflect people's lived experience in most communities around the world. One of the effects of this ontology has been to obscure the particular experiences of women, who are most likely to define themselves in and through their relations with children and other family members – including the elderly or chronically ill – or with friends or members of their communities. This is not to say that the picture of "autonomous man" distorts only the experiences of women; indeed, care ethicists argue that all people live lives that are, at least during some periods of time, interdependent with those of others and that moral analysis must reflect, rather than obscure, this fundamental characteristic of human existence.

The second feature of care ethics – the focus on responsibilities to particular others – is among the most controversial. This can be explained in two ways. First, the hostility to this view of ethics arises from the dominance of traditional approaches to ethics, which call for impartiality and universality in moral thinking and which rely on the application of abstract rules to particular moral situations. Morality is said to demand that the moral agent be able to remove him/herself from the emotional, private feelings that are seen to characterize our responses in the context of personal relationships; indeed, the highest stage of morality is seen to be characterized by a morality of rationality that can apply principles without bias. As Tronto (1993, 13) argues, this kind of approach to ethics presumes that we think most clearly about others when we think of them as distant from us. "Closeness" is seen to lead to "clouded" moral thinking and, ultimately, to partiality, favouritism, and nepotism.

This argument, however, relies on a caricature of care ethics as counselling that moral attention should be bestowed on those "near and dear" or, worse, those who are in some ways "like" us. No existing version of care ethics argues this; rather, care ethicists argue that people experience their moral lives in the context of webs of relationships with individuals and groups of particular others and that one of the main tasks of moral inquiry is to think about how care, and responsibilities for care, is distributed both within and across societies. This does not preclude concern for distant others or those who are not "like" us; on the contrary, as I discuss below, this approach actually offers us resources with which to evaluate critically dominant moral understandings.

The other source of hostility towards the particularism of care ethics comes from the frequent invocation of the mother-child relationship as paradigmatic of this approach to morality. This has been wrongly interpreted as suggesting that there is a natural or essential link between women's identity and motherhood or of idealizing the mother-child relationship as morally superior and, thus, ignoring the conflict, power imbalances, indifference, and even cruelty that can potentially characterize it. This reading ignores the fact that those who use this example – including Virginia Held and Sara Ruddick – do so in order to provide a *model* of moral reasoning from which important moral values can be derived (see Held 1993; Ruddick 1989).

That said, there may be other problems with relying too heavily on the mother-child model. As Selma Sevenhuijsen (1998, 13) argues, associating the "mother figure" with values such as concreteness, care, and compassion as opposed to abstraction and justice runs the risk of reproducing the mode of arguing in binary oppositions, with which Western thinking is so thoroughly permeated. Moreover, this model may serve to direct attention away from the political aspects of care and the more basic questions of the quality of moral identities and moral subject positions that feminists construct in their reasoning (ibid.).

The third feature of care ethics – the commitment to context – is clearly related to the previous two ideas. To quote Sevenhuijsen again, the moral agent in an ethics of care stands "with both feet in the real world"; this is in contrast to the ideal moral agent of universalist ethics, which must abstract from specific circumstances in order to achieve responsible moral judgment. On this view, situatedness in concrete social practices is not a threat to independent judgment; indeed, the ethics of care demands reflection on the best course of action in specific circumstances (Sevenhuijsen 1998, 59). Moreover, as Eva Kittay argues, there appear to be universal aspects of the meaning and experience of caring, including, at a most basic level, that it is required by all human beings at some time in their lives. However, differences in ability, race, gender, sexuality, religion, culture, and geography orient us differently towards care, making questions concerning the giving and receiving of care a matter of social, moral, and political import (Kittay 2005, 444-45).

Finally, the ethics of care must be committed to a radical reconceptualization of the public/private dichotomy – especially as it has developed in Western societies and "international society" through the legacy of Western liberalism. This means a rethinking of the nature of public and private as it relates to ethics. In particular, it must challenge the assertion by a number of prominent male moral and political philosophers that care matters in the context of intimate, personal relationships but that it is irrelevant, or dangerous, in the "real" context of ethics – the public realm. Challenging this account of public and private ethics must be part of a wider contestation of what counts as political and how these assumptions are fundamentally constituted through historically constructed gender norms, roles, and power relations.

While the earliest work on care ethics concentrates on care as an alternative to justice as a form of moral reasoning, later works seek to interrogate the political implications of care (Tronto 1993; Sevenhuijsen 1998). More recently, research on care ethics and care work has begun to explore care in a global context (Robinson 1999, 2006b; Held 2006; Porter 2006; Lawson 2007). In 2006, Elizabeth Porter (2006, 99) argued that there has been minimal application of the themes of care ethics to political issues in international relations, where the care of distant humans is paramount.[1] Her article goes on to elaborate on a "politics of care" and a "politics of compassion," where the latter links the universal and the particular in that it "assumes a shared humanity of interconnected, vulnerable people and requires emotions and practical, particular responses to different expressions of vulnerability" (Porter 2006, 99). Similarly, in *The Ethics of Care: Personal, Political, and Global,* Virginia Held (2006, 155) suggests that the ethics of care is "beginning to influence how those interested in international relations and global politics see the world and our responsibilities in it, and it holds promise for new efforts to improve global relations." Like Porter, she argues that a global ethics of care can be constructed in order to extend caring moral responses beyond the realm of private or personal relationships to the global context.

While there is widespread agreement among feminist ethicists and political philosophers regarding the substantive characteristics of care ethics – that is, relational ontology and the substantive features of ethics that flow from that – there is rather less agreement regarding epistemological and methodological questions in care ethics. Care ethicists – and feminist moral philosophers more broadly – have differing views on epistemology and, specifically, the nature and status of moral judgment in the ethics of care, the "form" of care ethics (as opposed to traditional moral theories), and the methods of moral inquiry that arise from a feminist ethics of care.

My own approach to these issues is informed by the work of Margaret Walker (1989, 21), who argues that, embedded within feminist ethics, are a number of "potent critical resources." These are of great significance to the construction of a critical feminist ethics of world politics: "The obvious ones I see are its structural capacity to challenge 'principled' moral stances in the concrete, where these are surrogates for, or defenses against, responsiveness in actual relationships; to export an insistence on the primacy of personal acknowledgement and communication to institutional and 'stranger' contexts; and on a philosophical plane to pierce through the rhetoric of ethics to the politics of ethics as a routine matter" (146). Eschewing epistemological foundationalism and moral universalism, Walker defends an epistemology that she defines as "naturalized" *and* "critical." The object of study is moral knowledge produced and sustained within communities. It has two tasks: "First, it must identify what kinds of things people need to know to live according to moral understandings that prevail in (any of) their possibly multiple communities or societies. And it must supply critical strategies and standards for testing whether understandings about how to live that are most credited in a community or society deserve their authority" (Walker 1998, 60). A critical feminist ethics of care seeks to interrogate how illusions of self-sufficiency – and the normative primacy attached to "autonomy" in most Western societies and through the institutions of global governance – are enabled and sustained by the undervalued and often unremunerated caring labour of the least advantaged members of society (often women of colour from income-poor countries). Thus, while it may seem that many men are autonomous, and that indeed many women in income-rich countries are increasingly autonomous, the apparent emancipation of these individuals is at the cost of the oppression – sometimes even enslavement – of others. This oppression is supported by the widespread degradation of caring roles; rather than being seen as empowering or as a valuable civic contribution requiring important skills, both givers and receivers of care are widely regarded as dependent and subservient.

Thus, a critical feminist ethics of care does not understand ethics as a set of principles waiting to be "applied" to a particular issue in world politics; rather, it views the task of normative or moral theory as one of *critical moral ethnography* – understanding how morality is "seated and reproduced in actual human societies" (Walker 1998, 211).[2] On this view, morality is not, as Walker says, "socially modular"; on the contrary, it is embedded within the social, material, and discursive hierarchies that characterize most societies. Thus, moral standards, statuses, and distributions of responsibility must be seen as working *through* social differences rather than in spite of them (ibid.). When "doing" ethics is understood in this way, it becomes clear that the moral theorist cannot choose to abstain from the work of *really looking* at social, economic, and political arrangements by claiming that they are not the stuff of moral theory.

Using a critical feminist ethics of care as a moral framework through which to view global care work and sex work shifts attention towards an examination of the wider context in which these activities take place. Furthermore, rather than regarding female care and sex workers, their employers, and their clients as autonomous individuals who either possess or lack agency to make moral decisions, a critical ethics of care regards all people as embedded within networks of relationships. Relative power, degrees of agency, and moral responses are mediated through these relationships. Some relationships may be nurturing and life-sustaining, while others may be exploitative or violent; good caring relations, however, are always vital for human security.[3]

Using this approach facilitates a critique of the stereotype of care as "bottomless feminine nurturance and self-sacrifice" (Walker 1998, 108). Critics of care ethics – including some feminists – argue that an ethics of care can serve to reinforce gender stereotypes and can "look like the lamentable internalization of an oppressively servile social role" (ibid.). That care has come to be degraded in this way, however, is a result of the development of particular moral understandings – including hegemonic forms of masculinity – that are mediated through gendered relations of power. As Jan Pettman argues, the domestication of women naturalizes men's sex right to women's bodies, labour, and children. Women are there to service men, providing domestic and sexual labour, which is assumed to be a labour of love (Pettman 1996, 186).

While there is no essential picture of what good caring relations should look like, a critical ethics of care emphasizes the benefits to all people of an image of care that recognizes responsibility and responsiveness to particular others as positive expressions of both masculinity and femininity. A critical feminist ethics must reclaim the role of caring values as a positive, valuable aspect of all societies and of caring labour as an important practice of contemporary citizenship. In the context of global politics, it asserts that the adequate provision of care, and equitable distribution of responsibilities for care, is a basic feature of global justice and human security.

Interrogating the Ethics of the Global Political Economy of Care: Hegemonic Masculinity and Gendered Globalization

While literature on care ethics has engaged extensively with "femininity" and the feminization of care, it has been relatively silent on masculinity and its relationship with the values and practices of caring.[4] Notions of masculinity and femininity are necessarily interdependent and intersect with other social relations of power, including race and class. While the language of care may be the "different voice" of women, a critical care ethics must eschew gender essentialisms and interrogate how hegemonic forms of masculinity license men's neglect of caring responsibilities and contribute to the manipulation of images of care and womanhood into images of female subservience and sexual service.

The concept of hegemonic masculinity is only about two decades old, but it has had a considerable influence on thinking and research on gender relations in a variety of contexts (Connell and Messerschmidt 2005, 829). Most important, the idea of hegemonic masculinity is able to explain how there could be multiple masculinities at a given time and how certain forms of masculinity could be more socially central, or more associated with authority and social power, than others. Moreover, the term "hegemonic" supports the idea that the hierarchy of masculinities is a pattern of hegemony, not a pattern of simple domination based on force. Thus, although they may only be enacted by a minority of "real" men, hegemonic masculinities are created and reinforced through cultural consent, discursive centrality, institutionalization, and the marginalization or delegitimation of alternatives (846).

Feminist analyses of global political economy demonstrate how cultures of hegemonic masculinity are integral to both the discursive and material constitution of globalization. As Charlotte Hooper (2000, 67-68) argues, the imagery of hegemonic masculinity positions globalization firmly in the "glamorous masculine conceptual space of the 'international', as far from the feminized world of domestic life as possible." She goes on: "It is 'out there' in the international arena which only intrepid businessmen fear to tread, as opposed to 'in here' in the domestic space of businessmen's homes where global restructuring has directed a tide of often illegal and under-age female migrants and domestic servants" (68).

Understanding the influence of hegemonic masculinities in the constitution of governance rules at global and national levels is crucial to an analysis of sex trafficking. Indeed, this can help to explain why these rules have yet to give due recognition to the significance of women's work relative to men's work, and of women's security needs relative to men's security needs. As Thanh-Dam Truong (2003, 32-33) argues, whereas care for the old, the sick, and the young – socially defined as women's work – tends to meet with less supportive responses from state-based and community-based entitlement systems, care for men's sexual needs is highly responsive to market forces.

Norms of hegemonic masculinities contribute to the feminizing of domestic, service, and sex work; in so doing, they serve to reify the public/private dichotomy and mute the contradictions of transnational liberalism (Chang and Ling 2000, 41). Just as the articulation of two separate spheres of human social life – the public and the private – served to obfuscate the gender contradictions of early liberal theories of rights, the "transnational ideology of sexualized, racialized service" allows the public, masculine face of globalization to flourish (ibid.). This "public" globalization – what Chang and Ling call "techno-muscular capitalism" – valorizes those norms and practices usually associated with Western capitalist masculinity but masked as global or universal. This face of globalization is supported and sustained by a "privatized" regime of "labour intimacy" – a sexualized, racialized, class-based regime of low-wage caring services provided by mostly female migrant workers (27). It is a feminized, privatized globalization that, although muted, is essential for the survival of both (1) the processes and practices of "techno-muscular capitalism" and (2) the reproduction of the moral understandings that legitimize and sustain them.

Contemporary forms of hegemonic masculinity are constructed through accounts of femininity as caring, docile, dependent, and self-sacrificing. Significantly, in the context of the sex trade, these accounts are also raced and thus construct this type of femininity as foreign, exotic, and "Other."[5] Here, relations of gender and race intersect. As Pettman (1996, 198) argues, in a postcolonial era, colonial relations live on in racialized power differences and intensifying relations of dominance, subordination, and exploitation.

While it is crucial to interrogate forms of masculinity and their relationship to norms and practices associated with caring, it is important to note that the transformation of masculinities must not be confined to the household or "intimate" level. In her study of the World Bank's efforts to resolve the "social reproduction dilemma" in Ecuador, Kate Bedford (2008) shows how the strategies employed – which focused on teaching men how to be responsible and reliable family members by increasing their participation in caring labour – resulted in the complete endorsement of privatized solutions to social reproduction, thus erasing child-care provision as a priority. While she acknowledges that the problems of male irresponsibility and violence are "very real," the discursive constructions of violent and lazy men in World Bank documents are both racialized and classed, and they are not supported by persuasive evidence (99).

The idea of hegemonic masculinities is not designed to describe the behaviour or activities of individual men. On the contrary, it describes a set of fluid, socially constructed norms about "maleness" that are constituted by and embedded within social structures and institutions. While there is certainly a relationship between these norms and the behaviour of some men some of the time, solutions to unequal or oppressive gender relations cannot focus on changing men's behaviour. Particular forms of masculinity must be recognized as constitutive of wider structures and institutions, including neoliberal development policies and "globalization" more generally as well as national and global cultures of militarism and military institutions. An important factor in shaping the visions of masculinity that constitute these structures and institutions is a vision of care as a private, feminine, low-value activity. These visions of masculinity will be transformed by focusing primarily not on the level of the household but, rather, on the institutions of global economic and security governance.

Sex Work and Care Work in the Global Political Economy

> *Sex service discourse is not so different from discourses on housework and caring, all trying to define tasks that can be bought and sold as well as assert a special human touch. Paid activities may include the production of feelings of intimacy and reciprocity, whether the individuals involved intend them or not, and despite the fact that overall structures are patriarchal and unjust.*
>
> – Laura Agustin (2007)

Unlike the global care economy, which is seen as morally unproblematic, the global sex economy is rife with moral discourse. Interestingly, there is little consensus regarding what constitutes the central ethical debates surrounding these practices. This is reflected in the priorities of various anti-sex trafficking groups, which identify trafficking as a problem for very different reasons and have very different political agendas with regard to the issue (O'Connell Davidson 2006, 7). Thus, for many states, the problem with sex trafficking arises out of issues concerning irregular immigration and transnational organized crime. For human rights NGOs, interest is often based on labour rights and concerns about "modern slavery" (8). For feminist abolitionist groups, often in coalition with groups from the religious right, prostitution and sex trafficking are condemned as a "social evil" that is asserted to be "immoral" in that it is oppressive and exploitative of women and/or a threat to marriage and the family (Weitzer 2007, 450). It is this group that makes use of the most explicitly "moral" language and that has constructed the fight against prostitution and sex trafficking as a moral crusade. The goals of a moral crusade, furthermore, are twofold. As Weitzer explains: "These movements ... see their mission as a righteous enterprise whose goals are both symbolic (attempting to redraw or bolster normative boundaries and moral standards) and instrumental (providing relief to victims, punishing evildoers)" (448). This kind of moral analysis – which relies on the rhetoric of "good" and "evil" and makes authoritative moral prescriptions about threats to moral and social fabric – fails to incorporate critical moral ethnography (which, I argue, is a crucial feature of feminist moral inquiry). As Walker (1998, 75) argues, it is a central work of feminist moral analysis to analyze the discursive spaces that different moral views (and theories of them) create and to explore the positions of agency and distributions of responsibility that these views foreground or eclipse. Significantly, moreover, it is important to look at where moral views are "socially sited" and what relations of authority and power hold them in place.

The moral crusades against prostitution and organized crime fail to understand prostitution and sex trafficking in the wider social-moral contexts of the transnationalization of women's sex and care work and the normative structures that uphold those processes. In particular, they obscure the extent to which the contemporary global migration and trafficking of women is anchored in particular features of the current globalization of economies in both the North and the South (Sassen 2002). The last decade has seen a growing number of women in a variety of cross-border circuits that have become a source for livelihood, profit-making, and the accrual of foreign currency (256). These developments can be seen as indicators of the "feminization of survival"; in other words, it is increasingly on the backs of low-wage and poor women that these forms of survival, profit-making, and government revenue enhancement operate (274). These global circuits tend to be concentrated in care work and intimate labour that is socially constructed as women's work – domestic labour, including housework and child care; nursing and care for the sick and the elderly; and sex work. Although unremunerated, the "work" of mail-order brides can be seen as part of these circuits in that the process of recruitment of brides and the contractual agreements between the parties is regulated and institutionalized by governments.[6]

A combination of economic, social, and demographic factors have led to the growth of "alternative circuits of survival in developing countries." These conditions include the effects of structural adjustment programs (SAPs) and the opening of economies to foreign firms. In turn, these conditions have given rise to a series of economic costs: unemployment, the closure of many firms in traditional sectors oriented to local markets, and the ongoing and increasing burden of government debt in most developing economies (Sassen 2002, 257). It is this "growing inmiseration" of governments and whole economies in the South that has "promoted and enabled the proliferation of survival and profit-making activities that involve the migration and trafficking of (low-wage and poor) women" (255).

In spite of discursive and policy efforts to separate "sex" workers from other forms of migrant female labour, all of this global women's work may be traced, in large measure, to the same norms and processes. As Audrey Macklin argues, there is a global demand for "women's work" that can no longer be supplied by women in affluent, developed states. While the types and nature of this work differ somewhat, all these forms of labour can only be made sense of when viewed through the lens of global gendered relations of power. Thus, as Macklin points out, sex-trade workers supply sex, live-in caregivers perform child care and housework, and so-called "mail-order brides" furnish all three. Yet, although sex-trade workers are "frequently criminalized as prostitutes and 'mail-order brides' are not formally designated as workers (insofar as their labour is unpaid), these migrations occur within a commercialized context where the expectation of economic benefit (to the women and to relatives in the country of origin) structures the incentives for entering the process" (Macklin 2003, 464-65).

One solution to the problem of separating sex workers from other types of workers is to address all of this work from within the framework of women's rights. For example, Christien van den Anker (2006, 180) points to the lack of integration between the discourse on migrant workers' rights and the discourse on women's rights, and argues that migrant women "should be an important part of the women's rights agenda" (180). She insists that, in spite of the fractured and legalistic nature of rights discourse and implementation, a rights approach is regarded as the best way to conceptualize, and potentially to transform, the problem of human trafficking. This is in line with the analytical and normative framework taken by many non-abolitionist feminists towards human trafficking (see Kempadoo 2005; Chang and Kim 2007; Van den Anker 2006) and towards gender and human security more broadly.

Clearly, rights-based ethics, rights discourse, and human rights law have a role to play in addressing the issue of sex trafficking, in both academic and activist contexts. This is especially the case when rights are seen as embedded within wider structures of globalization and so-called "root causes." As Van den Anker (2006, 179) argues, "gender, race, nationality and ethnicity are at least some of the factors influencing who ends up trafficked and under which circumstances. Universalist approaches therefore need to take into account that these structural and long-term causes may need recognition before equal respect can be implemented" (ibid.). On this view, rights are not seen as abstract or ahistorical but, rather, as situated within the gendered effects of globalization and framed by an intersectional approach.

While this kind of women's rights approach to sex trafficking moves in the right direction – in terms of its commitment to situating trafficking within gendered globalization – it is destined always to see trafficking as a women's rights "issue" and, thus, of relevance only to women. It is also likely to remain plagued by debates over universality and difference – especially among so-called "First World" and "Third World" women. Furthermore, a rights-based approach cannot give us insight into *why and how* these abuses are licensed by dominant social and cultural norms or "moral understandings." A critical feminist ethics of care, by contrast, helps us to understand the designation and assignment of "women's work" and the subsequent feminization and devaluation of the values and practices of care.

Conclusion: Reclaiming Care

In this chapter, I argue that normative analyses of "women's work" in the global economy – especially domestic, care, and sex work – require engaging in a "critical moral ethnography" in order to uncover the moral understandings that license and legitimize the flourishing global care and sex economies. Such an approach to ethics requires seeing these moral understandings as embedded within the structures and processes of the gendered global political economy. The prevalence of these forms of labour in the contemporary global economy demonstrate how the values and practices of care have been denigrated and manipulated by unequal power relations of gender and race as well as by wider inequalities in the global political economy.

The naturalized epistemology of critical feminist care ethics offers no obvious moral or policy prescriptions. It does, however, start with some clear ontological arguments about relationality and the life-sustaining significance of caring relations and caring responsibilities for all human flourishing. It regards these relations and responsibilities as neither "natural" nor "contractual" but as fundamentally ethical. As such, they are inseparable from, and indeed are constituted by, the social, economic, and political arrangements within which they are embedded in household, local, and global contexts. Furthermore, arrangements for care in particular contexts may be judged "better" or "worse": they may be characterized by inequalities, exploitation, oppression, or by fairness, transparency, trust, and equity. Responsibilities for care may be gendered and raced or they may be distributed fairly, based on the assumption that all persons are bearers of responsibilities to care for others; access to care from others may be unequal or it may be available to all persons.

Current trends of globalization – specifically, the sexualization and commodification of female migrant labour within peripheral sites and the accelerating exchange of money for bodies – are part of wider trends towards neoliberal restructuring that contribute to the socio-economic and political conditions that feminize, racialize, denigrate, and undervalue the activities of care. Rather than being upheld as a fundamental, life-sustaining activity of citizenship, care is associated with subservience, self-sacrifice, dependence, and a lack of agency. Care work, domestic work, and sex work – increasingly undertaken by migrant women of colour – occupy the lowest rungs on the ladder of "success" in the global political economy. Often alone and "out of place," the women who perform this work are, ironically, highly vulnerable in terms of their lack of relationship networks, family, and formal citizenship status. Thus, these "foreign" carers are perhaps the least likely to receive good care, and many lead lives that are perpetually insecure.

While changes in policy at the level of state welfare regimes and international financial institutions are crucial, some change to local and global notions of masculinity and femininity are necessary if real transformation to the global organization of care, and the nature of "women's work" more generally, is to take place. In her analysis of the global "sex economy," Thanh-Dam Truong (2003) argues that cultural means must be found to deal with forms of expression of masculinity that are harmful to the integrity of women and children as social beings. Current expressions of masculinity in the sex trade need to be countered with "images of virility as the ability to care and take responsibility for the other" (48). She argues for a notion of "caring and responsible" sex (as distinct from "safe sex") that seeks not only to enhance personal safety but also to promote a cultural transformation towards non-violence in sexuality. It is through non-violence, she argues, that mutual respect can be built and a gender-based human security achieved (ibid.). As I have argued, however, it is crucial that efforts to transform sexuality and, in particular, masculinity are not directed towards particular men or individual households; on the contrary, cultures of masculinity cannot be divorced from the wider institutions and structures of global governance that are themselves constituted through gender relations and particular understandings of masculinity and femininity – including an understanding of care as a private, feminine, low-value activity.

Moreover, attempts to define what masculinity or sexuality should "look like" are problematic and may lead back to the same "moralizing" debates that continue to dominate the ethical discussion of prostitution and sex trafficking. I would argue, in contrast, for a broad reanalysis of the role of care in societies – both domestically and at the level of "global society." This involves understanding how "new geographies of inequality" have simultaneously made care a more pressing concern and marginalized it (Lawson 2007, 2). Unlike a women's rights approach, a critical care ethics approach can help us to understand *why* women are economically and physically exploited and subject to violence through elucidating the connections between femininity and subservience, on the one hand, and masculinity and autonomy, on the other. Shifts in moral understandings towards the valuing of care and the reshaping of visions of masculinity and femininity must go hand in hand with the recognition of care as the very basis of active citizenship and human security.

8

The Dark Side of Care
The Push Factors of Human Trafficking

OLENA HANKIVSKY

Sex trafficking, which disproportionately affects women, has garnered significant political attention and has prompted the development of a range of anti-trafficking international rules and domestic laws. While increasing emphasis is being paid to exploring the underlying causes that prompt women from developing and transitional countries to seek alternative livelihoods abroad, few analyses have explicitly recognized, as does this chapter, caring motivations as fundamental to seeking out such opportunities, which often place women in oppressive and dangerous situations. Many women who seek employment abroad and then become victims of sex trafficking seek to improve levels of well-being for their families, including their children. Unlike many other forms of international labour, however, the coercive nature of sex trafficking often prevents women from sending any remittances to family members in home countries. Moreover, because of the threats made by traffickers towards their families and children, women who are trafficked into the sex trade also resist fleeing or reporting on their experiences.

In this chapter, I draw on care ethics to challenge traditional explanations of push and pull factors and argue that an incomplete understanding of these, especially the push factors, impedes adequate policy responses to sex trafficking. In so doing, I build on recent work by care scholars who interrogate care in the global context (Tronto 2008; Held 2006; Hankivsky 2006); in particular, I draw on the work of Fiona Robinson who, most recently, examines the relevance of care in the area of human security (2008a) and sex trafficking (2008b). While Robinson (2008b) argues that a critical, feminist ethics of care can provide a comprehensive ontological and normative framework for reconceptualizing human security and the demand side of sex trafficking, in what follows, I describe how care ethics can deepen the understanding of the root causes of migration and, in the process, provide insights into a largely uninvestigated dimension of transnational sex trafficking – female migrant responses to "care deficits."

I begin with an introduction to the definition and conceptualization of migration and sex trafficking. I then move on to consider Ukraine, one of the most seriously affected countries. In so doing, I argue that economic circumstances and the poverty of individual women are typically highlighted as the key explanatory reasons that women seek opportunities abroad, without taking into account the way these are linked to caregiving identities, roles, and responsibilities. Moreover, by drawing on the values of care, including contextual sensitivity, responsiveness (which includes drawing on narratives and stories of women survivors), and consequences of policy decisions, I reveal the importance of care ethics for expanding on current understandings of and potential responses to sex trafficking. I argue that what is often missing as an explicit dimension in the analysis of push factors in migration and sex trafficking is attention to the human and political consequences of the fundamental human need for care, especially when this need becomes impossible for caregivers and care receivers to fulfill or to realize. I conclude with some directions on how attention to the values associated with care ethics can inform interventions that are better tailored to reduce and respond to the problem of sex trafficking not only in Ukraine but also in other jurisdictions.

Migration and Trafficking

Migration can be understood as the "general movement of people who voluntarily or forcedly leave their homes in search of a better life" (Levchenko and Shvab 2008, 7). While not all migrants are victims of trafficking, many migrants hoping to improve their socio-economic status end up in the hands of traffickers, who exploit them, hold them in oppressive slave-like conditions, and treat them in a cruel and inhuman manner. Trafficking can therefore be understood as a distorted mode of migration (UNICEF et al. 2005). According to the UN Convention against Transnational Organized Crime's protocol, trafficking in persons may be defined as:

The recruitment, transportation, transfer, harbouring or receipt of persons, by means of the threat or use of force or other forms of coercion, of abduction, of fraud, of deception, of the abuse of power or of a position of vulnerability or of the giving or receiving of payments or benefits to achieve the consent of a person having control over another person, for the purposes of exploitation. Exploitation shall include, at a minimum, the exploitation or the prostitution of others or other forms of sexual exploitation, forced labour or services, slavery or practices similar to slavery, servitude or the removal of organs. (United Nations 2000, Article 3)

The International Labour Organization estimates that, at any given time, there are 12.3 million people in forced labour, bonded labour, forced child labour, and sexual servitude. Furthermore, the organization estimates that sex trafficking yields profits amounting to $217.8 billion a year, or $23,000 per victim (US Department of State 2008, 36). Beyond these profits, however, is the human cost of trafficking – the physical and emotional abuse, rape, threats against self and family, and even death experienced by its victims. Approximately 80 percent of transnational victims are women and girls, and up to 50 percent are minors, many of whom fall victim to sex trafficking. Although the problem of sex trafficking arguably affects the health, safety, and security of all nations that are touched by this growing problem, there are particular countries that stand out, most notably those of the former Soviet Union – Moldova, Russia, and Ukraine.

Case Study: Ukraine and Sex Trafficking

As a country of origin and transit point, Ukraine has one of the worst human trafficking records in Europe. Since the collapse of the Soviet Union, more men, women, and children from Ukraine have been trafficked abroad and forced into indentured labour or prostitution than from any other Eastern European country. The majority of those affected are women, trafficked into the sex trade in countries such as Russia, Poland, Turkey, the Czech Republic, the United Arab Emirates, Austria, Italy, Portugal, Germany, Greece, Israel, Spain, Lebanon, Hungary, the Slovak Republic, Cyprus, the United Kingdom, the Netherlands, Serbia, Argentina, Norway, and Bahrain. According to an International Organization for Migration survey released in 2006, since 1991, approximately 117,000 Ukrainians have been forced into exploitative situations in Europe, the Middle East, and Russia (quoted in US Department of State 2008).

The extent of the problem has drawn international attention. The Ukrainian government – along with several NGOs – has attempted to respond to the issue, taking concrete steps to improve the status of women, reverse the emigration of women, and combat trafficking (for more detailed discussion of developments, see Hankivsky 2008; Pyshchulina 2005). Nevertheless, despite its efforts to date, Ukraine is routinely evaluated as not fully complying with the minimum standards for the elimination of trafficking (US State Department of State 2010). In 2010 the State Department recommended that Ukraine "seek sentences for convicted trafficking offenders that require them to serve appropriate jail time; continue to monitor human trafficking trial procedures and encourage prosecutors to give more serious attention to human trafficking cases by appealing non-custodial sentences; vigorously investigate and prosecute trafficking complicity by government officials; continue to take steps to establish formal mechanisms for the proactive identification and referral of trafficking victims to services; increase funding for NGOs providing critical care to victims; consider establishing a fund derived from assets seized from convicted traffickers for this purpose; provide specialized assistance to child trafficking victims; and continue trafficking-specific training for prosecutors and judges" (US Department of State 2010, 332). For the most part, the country's internal responses have been ineffectual, and inadequate attention has been paid to addressing the root causes of, and the vulnerabilities to, trafficking, which encompass myriad push and pull factors. In particular, the full range of factors that contribute to the willingness of women to risk trafficking remain largely uninvestigated (Hankivsky 2008; Rohatynskyj 2003).

"Push and Pull"

The importance of understanding the root causes of human trafficking has been emphasized in the literature, particularly in the context of the Commonwealth of Independent States (CIS) region. As explained by the UNDP (2007a, 7): "Trafficking in human beings in the CIS region can be viewed as the extreme expression of socio-economic and institutional breakdown and inequality in Eastern Europe and the CIS. The social and economic decline in the region, as well as the prospects of work in Western Europe, has, in the context of restricted migration, given traffickers' room to exploit individuals." More specifically, according to the UNDP (2007a), poverty, which is marked by the lack of access to development resources, including decent employment, education, health, and social protection, increases one's risk of being trafficked.

The growth of human and, specifically, sex trafficking is due to the social, political, and economic factors that push people from one country to another and pull them towards more prosperous, often Western, countries. Globalization has been central to these phenomena, through the opening of borders, the rise of international criminal network groups, and growing inequities between regions and among countries. The desire to move to a Western country to take up employment that promises "quick money earnings" (Winrock International 2001) has been pervasive within CIS countries since the breakdown of the Soviet Union, despite fairly tight restrictions on mobility. Also influential has been the "myth of an easy and affluent life in the West" (Pyshchulina 2005, 116). For example, in 1991, independence for Ukraine brought unprecedented hope for the future of the country. Nevertheless, political, economic, and social transitions have been slow and uneven, prompting a significant number of citizens to seek out opportunities abroad. Compared to other former Soviet countries, Ukraine lags behind in terms of political and economic reforms (116). An estimated 45 percent of the population currently lives on under four dollars per day (UNDP 2007b). The World Bank-estimated average annual purchasing power of Ukrainians is $7,000 per person, compared to $46,000 in the United States. The economy continues to fail, there is virtually no sense of job security, and the long and ongoing transition to a market economy has not been accompanied by attention to the social fabric of society or to the maintenance of a viable social welfare system. In response, many Ukrainians are seeking work abroad. Estimates report that 2 to 7 million Ukrainians reside and work abroad (Lutz 2008). While working abroad can contribute "to the growth, expertise, activity level, and well-being ensuring inflow of foreign currency" (Levchenko and Shvab 2008, 4), it has negative consequences, especially when workers fall victim to the human and sex trafficking industry. Most such victims are women.

The fact that most victims of trafficking are women is not altogether surprising as the period of "transition" in Ukraine has had particularly negative consequences for the female population. The UNDP (2007a, 7) effectively summarizes the disparate gendered effects of political, economic, and social change in all CIS countries, including Ukraine, in the following:

> The changes strengthened the patriarchal attitudes towards gender roles and increased the differences in the status of men and women. There is widespread discrimination against women in the labour market in terms of access to well-paid jobs as well as lower level of pay. As a result, women are

less competitive in the labour market and occupy a substantially lower position in the area of employment than men, even if the two have similar social and professional characteristics. While there is clearly discrimination against women in access to decision-making and employment, the general indicators of poverty are very similar for men and women.[1] However, poverty is high among specific groups of women, including older women of pension age, divorced or widowed women and women raising children alone. There is also a phenomenon of women with children falling into poverty after their husband/father has migrated for work.

After the collapse of the Soviet Union, unemployment hit women particularly hard: in Ukraine, 80 percent of all unemployed are women (Pyshchulina 2005). This is the result not only of changing economic circumstances but also of growing discrimination against and harassment of women in the workplace (Hankivsky and Salnykova, forthcoming). Moreover, the burden of transitioning to a market economy has weighed more heavily on women than on men, particularly because of the decline and or elimination of key health, social, and public services occurring alongside growing unemployment and higher inflation. For instance, many women find themselves sole breadwinners in their families, a responsibility complicated by the fact that public child-care centres have closed in great numbers. The collapse of social infrastructure and the loss of child-care facilities have led to increasing difficulties for families and particularly for women as they still bear the main responsibility for child care (UNICEF et al. 2005). Finally, as is the pattern in many other countries of the world, women often find themselves responsible not only for the care of their immediate families but also for the care of their elderly parents and extended relatives.

The net effect of such changes is that 65 percent of all migrants from Ukraine are women (Kyzyma 2007). Many of these women are at risk for sex trafficking. This is substantiated by La Strada, the key NGO working to prevent trafficking in women and helping the victims of trafficking in Ukraine:

> The most serious internal factors are rooted in Ukraine's poor economic situation, which has resulted for many in the inability to find adequate employment – and a lack of viable alternatives for earning money. The problem is especially significant when it comes to Ukrainian women ... [because] the feminization of poverty has led to a situation where women are desperate to find work and may fail to consider the possible negative consequences attached to some offers. (Jones 2005, 2)

Economic conditions and concomitant poverty in Ukraine are thus cited as the key reasons for the declining standard of living for Ukrainian women (Lakiza-Sachuk 2003), migration motivations, and the related risks of sex trafficking (Hankivsky 2008). Rohatynskyj (2003, 162) goes so far as to argue that "the willingness to entertain the possibility of the commodification of sexual services can be seen as an indication of what can be called the latest cultural hegemony to manifest itself through the Ukrainian population typified by aspirations to individual consumerism." This view, which is arguably consistent with the normative values of liberalism, sees human behaviour as linked to the rational pursuit of self-interest and optimal economic results (Hankivsky 2004). Rohatynskyj further asserts that "the logic of consumerism, unchecked by a countervailing social ethic, renders all goods, persons and services commodities" (163). This is consistent with Robinson and Mahon's (this volume) observation that the commodification of care, for example, is part of a wider trend towards the (gendered) commodification of all "intimate" services at the transnational level.

There is absolutely no doubt that the desire to improve socio-economic circumstances is a key factor in women's increasing willingness to risk a potentially dangerous situation in the web of global sex trafficking. What is missing from this explanatory framework, however, is a full recognition of relationality and an understanding that economic deprivation and poverty are experienced by individuals who are deeply embedded within human relations in which persons have a range of "responsibilities and need for care" (Robinson 2008a, 183). As Kempadoo, Sanghera, and Pattanaik (2005, xi) point out: "although many women are indeed coerced and violated in the global sex trade, their situations are in many ways similar to those of other migrant women who seek to make a livelihood for themselves and their families in a highly gendered and racialized world order." Those who leave are therefore motivated not only by consumerism or a self-maximizing need to improve their own lives but also by the "countervailing ethic" of care. Seen in this way, the ethics of care provides a critical lens through which to view sex trafficking. This lens enables us to understand more fully the push factors of sex trafficking as it views all human beings as existing within interdependent relations and, thus, as often prioritizing choices that preserve and protect those relations.

Care Ethics, Migration, and Sex Trafficking

Joan Tronto firmly establishes care's importance as *both* a moral and a political concept. It can be defined as a "species activity that includes everything that we do to maintain, continue and repair our 'world' so that we can live in it as well as possible. That world includes our bodies, our environments, all of which we seek to interweave in a complex, life-sustaining web" (Tronto 1993, 103). A more recent definition by Daniel Engster (2005, 55) posits that "caring may be said to include everything we do directly to help others to meet their basic needs, develop or sustain their basic capabilities, and alleviate or avoid pain or suffering, in an attentive, responsive and respectful manner." Engster further explains that "it is not just that we have depended and probably will depend someday upon the care of others, it is that human life is deeply implicated in relations of dependency and caring" (61). Similarly, in the context of international relations, "care ethics also reminds us that all people exist in webs of relations with others, and rely on those others for their care, and hence their security" (Robinson 2008b, 4). Within those relationships, each human being's subjective experience is created at the intersection of social locations determined by variables such as gender, socio-economic class, and geography.

Care ethics has a number of key defining features, effectively summarized by Robinson (2008b, 7): "An ethics of care includes the following: a relational ontology, which conceptualizes the selves as fully relational – existing in and through complex, constitutive webs or relations with others; a focus on attention, responsiveness and responsibility to the needs of particular others as core substantive moral values; a commitment to addressing moral problems in the historical and spatial contexts of real, lived experiences; and finally, a reconceptualization of traditional understandings of the nature of and relationship between the 'public' and 'private' spheres." Moreover, the normative criteria of care ethics, which I identify in early writings – namely, contextual sensitivity, responsiveness, and attention to the consequences of choice (Hankivsky 2004) – can alter the conceptualization of sex trafficking. Such an understanding of the centrality of caring in human lives can be applied not only to illuminate largely overlooked motivating factors for migration and susceptibility to sex trafficking but also to provide the basis for rethinking and transforming how governments and other institutions respond to this global problem.

Contextual Sensitivity

From the perspective of a care ethic, contextual sensitivity to the lives of women who experience sex trafficking is paramount. Using a critical feminist ethics of care as a moral framework through which to view sex trafficking shifts attention from individual or criminal behaviour towards an examination of the wider context in which these activities take place (Robinson 2008b, 10). This entails taking into account the political instability, socioeconomic situation, and deterioration of basic health and social systems and services in Ukraine. Particular attention needs to be paid to the financial and material challenges faced by many Ukrainian families and in circumstances that involve generally increasing social and emotional vulnerability (Tolstokorova 2009). Such an approach would account for the changing role and responsibilities of women in Ukrainian society. As noted above, the number of families in which women are the primary breadwinners is growing (Jones 2005), and 89 percent of the poorest families in Ukraine are headed by single mothers (UNICEF et al. 2005). Research has shown that, in the present context, Ukrainians report that citizens feel unable to improve their lives (Abbott and Wallace 2007); in the case of single mothers, this situation is exacerbated, as many find it impossible to deal with their family responsibilities. Not surprisingly, then, the "feminization of survival" (Sassen 2002) is often manifest in women moving across borders to make a living and, in many instances, attempting to remit their earnings home. It is important, however, to highlight that this feminization of survival is deeply embedded in complex, constitutive webs or relations with others, which include relations with immediate and extended family members (Sassen 2002).

Thus, while economic factors are consistently cited as primary reasons for seeking opportunities abroad, dominant discourses do not always highlight all the dimensions of female migrant lives. In a recent study on female migration in Ukraine, Kyzyma (2007) develops a portrait of a "typical" Ukrainian female migrant as a woman between the ages of twenty and twenty-nine who lives in a city in the western part of Ukraine, is married, and has at least one child (Kyzyma 2007). Others offer different types of profiles, especially with regard to trafficked women. For example, a 2002 Environmentally and Socially Sustainable Development (ECSSD) study finds that the majority of women who are trafficked are rural residents, have some form of secondary school education, and are over the age of twenty-five. Moreover, it finds that "many had been unable to find work, had children to support, and had left their children with relatives or friends when they sought work abroad" (Dudwick, Srinivasan, and Braithwaite 2002, 57).

The majority of female migrants, including those who may find themselves in the sex-trafficking industry, may differ in terms of geography, age, and education, but they are often similar in that they are mothers. In a recent survey of Ukrainian migrants in Italy, 75 percent of women reported leaving behind one or two children, while 8 percent left three or more. According to Kyzyma (2007, 10), "90% of female migrants have at least one child." Clearly, in the realm of policy, it may not be possible for all individual particularities to be captured. That said, it is worth noting that, in this instance, these women all have specific caregiving responsibilities to immediate family members (e.g., children) and, in many other instances, have direct responsibility for extended family members as well. This reality, combined with ever-decreasing economic security, makes it virtually impossible for many female citizens of Ukraine to sustain human life through care work. In this way, contextual sensitivity is effective in raising political questions about what needs exist, how they are being taken care of (or not), under what circumstances, and by whom.

Responsiveness

Subjective experiences, relayed through first- or third-person narratives, allow for traditionally marginalized and silenced voices to be heard; for knowledge to be gained about the nature of human needs, dependencies, and vulnerabilities; and (possibly) for the promotion of action to address these (Hankivsky 2004). Bruckert and Parent (2002, 12) are correct in observing that allowing "victims no voice to explain the meaning of their actions greatly reduces the scope of the problem of trafficking in humans." At the same time, for the most part, this population tends to be hidden in order to avoid stigmatization from communities and families or retribution from former traffickers. Most of the available information on the experience of being trafficked comes from women who return home, come forward, and seek assistance rather than from those who cannot return. In terms of the stories that have been made public, a common feature is the centrality of care practices – both the inability to care well in their present circumstances and the desperate need, driven by the responsibility to provide such care, to find a way to overcome the factors that impede it.

For a typical Ukrainian female migrant, including those who find themselves trafficked, seeking employment abroad is motivated by a number of factors, including: trying to find ways to respond to the various needs of their families (such as supporting parents and children) (Shapkina 2008); securing a better life for their families (Winrock International 2001); covering a child's education (Levchenko et al. 2010; Levchenko and Bandurko 2006), including university tuition (Kyzyma 2007); and improving the future for their children, including constructing and buying a home for their children (Levchenko and Schvab 2008; Levchenko and Bandurko 2006). It is estimated that remittances from Ukrainians working abroad total between US$4-6 billion annually, although, because of their slave-like existence, women who fall victim to sex trafficking rarely send any money home (Malynovska 2009).

Nevertheless, the risks associated with migration, including sex trafficking, do not seem to be deterrents. As Cherepakha, from the international women's right centre La Strada, explains, women are drawn to accepting "dubious" proposals to provide for families.[2] This is supported by numerous third-person accounts of survivors' experiences, a select few of which are highlighted below:

> Tanja lived in a small town in Lugansk region. She was 20 years old. Her father left the family when she was 4 and her brother was 2 years old. In 1991 her brother was run over by car. He stayed alive but became disabled. His mother couldn't work because she had to take care of him. Tanja graduated from a technical school but couldn't find work. No factories and plants in the city could offer employment. Sometimes the family had nothing to eat except bread and water. A friend of her mother proposed to her to go to her relatives in the United Arab Emirates and to work as a housemaid at a rich villa. The salary was US$4,000. It seemed incredible luck to the girl. She got the passport and visa and flew to Abu-Dhabi. (Levchenko 1999, 12)

> Marika was the perfect dupe. She was desperate for work. Her mother was sick and her father was an unemployed, miserable drunk. Her two younger sisters were wasting away. The job offer was her only chance to make things better. (Devas 2007)

> Svetlana and Oksana have been living together since childhood; they studied together and were great friends. After finishing school, Svetlana entered a culinary technical school, graduated and found a job [as] a cook in a canteen. As for Oksana, after finishing school she started working in a footwear workshop. But nevertheless the quantity of money they earned was not enough. Svetlana's mother was ill [and] that's why it was necessary to buy medicines ... Oksana divorced and was living alone with a little child. These situations made the girls look for additional jobs. (Cherepakha, author interview, 2009)

Stories that highlight the frustration of not being able to meet the demands of dependents are also highlighted in first-person narrative accounts:

I divorced my husband. There was not much support available, and I needed money. My parents are old. I have a child. When I got divorced, we had only my mom's income and that was not enough. (Woman survivor, in Shapkina [2008, 22])

My father has a sick heart, the doctors said he needed an operation. I worked at a bar but the money was not enough for such an operation. One day an acquaintance at the bar made me a job offer in Israel. It was in the sex trade. For two months I did not agree to it. But the acquaintance told me that that type of work in Israel is legal and that I would have security, an apartment, [a] mobile phone and that I could speak to my family on a regular basis and return home if I wanted. I finally agreed. (Survivor getting help from La Strada, Cherepakha, author interview, 2009)

I know one woman who says that she does not care that she had to sell sex because she brought money to her child. (Shapkina 2008, 99)

In addition, according to an Odessa focus group participant who took part in a study involving sex-trafficking survivors: "Women are motivated by the financial position of their families. Cases are not rare when a woman is the sole wage earner having to support her husband, child and the elderly mother. To this end, she is prepared even to sell her body. So, they take such jobs knowingly" (Dudwick, Srinivasan, and Braithwaite 2002, 56). Similarly, a woman survivor reports: "There was one woman who said that her child, for seven days, ate only apples. She stole those apples at night. And she decided to become a prostitute. She went abroad, and she was sold" (Shapkina 2008, 129).

Of course, these circumstances are not unique to the Ukrainian context: they also characterize the lives of women internationally who are, by a combination of factors, inextricably linked to their complex web of interdependent relations. As evidenced by the following two narratives, originally collected by StoptheTraffik.org, these women are at risk:

Sokha and Makara are from Poipet in Cambodia. When they were just 14 and 15 years old, their mother was ill with a liver complaint. The family needed money to pay for drugs to treat her. They also hoped to buy some land to build a home. A man promised good jobs for the girls in nearby Thailand, and offered the family some money if they would let them go. Sokha and Makara were excited at the thought of being able to help the family with the money they earned. The reality turned out to be very different. The man was a trafficker. There were no "good jobs" for the girls in Thailand. Sokha's mother died within a year, and the family couldn't afford to buy the land that they had dreamed of. Sokha, who is now 17, says, "I felt cheated. The traffickers used us for slave jobs, and while they earned lots of money, we only got enough to feed ourselves each day." (Kloer 2009)

In the words of a Thai woman trafficked to Japan:

I was told by an acquaintance to work at his restaurant in Japan. I decided to accept his offer as I thought my family might improve their life if I sent them my salary. Soon after my arrival in Japan, I realized that I was sold. My life since then has been like that of an animal. (Skrobanek 1998)

Once entrapped in the sex industry, women have very few exit options as they endure violence, rape, threats to themselves and their families, and debt bondage. For those women who do find a way to return home, only 12 percent report their victimization (Hughes and Denisova 2001). Many victims are unaware of their rights and are fearful of the traffickers, who are often local and know the victims' families. As explained by one survivor, "'If you will write [testimony], it is going to be worse for you, you will go to jail,' he said. He was threatening to kill me and my child. I was afraid, and I thought I should not go to police." For these kinds of reasons, many victims do not prosecute the traffickers, especially if they feel the latter will not be detained (Shapkina 2008, 47).

Consequences of Policy Choices: Moving Forward with New Understandings of Migration and Sex Trafficking

A recent UNDP report, *Trafficking in human beings in the Commonwealth of Independent States*, concludes that existing anti-trafficking approaches within the region are aimed at battling the consequences rather than the causes of the problem. According to the report, the root causes of trafficking in human beings are an integral part of the socio-economic structures and institutions that developed in the CIS region during the period of transition. The report concludes that, "without addressing the underlying causes, including mass poverty and limited access to development resources; the demand for cheap unprotected labour built into the CIS model of economic growth and the huge shadow economy that drives this demand; and the lack of access to safe and legal economic migration, human trafficking will continue to flourish" (UNDP 2007b, 14). While these are important observations, they do not tell the whole story. Migration and trafficking are not only linked to political transition, economic restructuring, and their resulting poverty, they are also part of what can be seen as a "crisis of care," that is, deep-seated care deficits that originate in the realm of the public sphere, through wrong-headed or inadequate policies that permeate the private sphere, making caring practices and responsibilities impossible to realize fully.

Care ethics is concerned with how "caring is enabled, sustained and protected" (Hutchings 2001, 209) across a number of realms and scales. As I argue elsewhere, "this can entail the proactive creation and maintenance of a progressive social safety net, one that permeates both the public and private realms, and one which ensures food and economic security, housing, health care, social assistance, education and adequate sanitation and facilitates support for a range of caregiving roles and responsibilities" (Hankivsky 2006, 98). While it must be acknowledged that, because of the way care is socially constructed and prescribed, the caregiving in any society is often disproportionately shouldered by women, it is also important to understand, as Robinson and Mahon (this volume) point out, that all citizens should have the right to give care on terms that reflect the value of the activity of caring. The ability to care, for oneself and for others, and to create and nurture caring practices can be seen as essential components of democratic citizenship. While it is true that caring motivations may be strongest within existing circles of interpersonal relations, the values of care ethics extend to all realms of the public sphere, including the transnational level.

Nevertheless, responses to sex trafficking do not recognize the links between care deficits and migration for economic purposes. For example, the Ukrainian state has not explicitly recognized the extent to which its economic reforms and related social policy changes have actually created structural barriers to enabling, sustaining, and protecting caring practices, including caregiving roles and responsibilities. Shapkina (2008, 31) similarly argues that, "by introducing economic reforms but failing to protect the well-being of the people and shield them from economic deprivation, the state contributed to the operation of sex trafficking markets." Rarely are economic reforms evaluated for their effects on the social fabric of society. From the perspective of care ethics, however, policies need to take into account the way economic reforms "would meet human needs and enable the care needed by all" (Held 2006, 152).

Ironically, many women in Ukraine and other countries who are trafficked for sex are shamed and vilified for "choosing" to abandon their countries, their families, and, especially, their children. While a number of studies examine the effects of female migration on families (Cherninska 2007; Yarova 2006), little attention is paid to the fact that, while many women can be seen as "choosing" to work abroad, these so-called choices are not always made under conditions of the women's own choosing (Shapkina 2008). The Ukrainian state and society, which historically and contemporarily prides itself on its "caring" relations, albeit from largely patriarchal perspectives in regard to the lives and well-being of women and children (Hankivsky and Salnykova, forthcoming; Dovzhenko 2001), has actually been instrumental in creating the conditions in which relations of care and care work are impossible to realize and migration becomes an imposed survival strategy. As Victor Malarek (2003, 2-3) describes in his investigative reporting: "With the social structure in disarray, families broke down. Children were abandoned on the street. Husbands sought solace in the bottle and alcoholism became an epidemic. Violence against women and children soared. And through it all, the women were left to pick up the pieces. They set out to find work to keep their families together. Even young girls with no families yet of their own went off searching for jobs to feed younger siblings and parents." Nevertheless, current public priorities in Ukraine – and also arguably across all international jurisdictions – tend not to reflect the integral role that care plays in our lives (Hankivsky 2004).

Thus, when analyzing the phenomenon of sex trafficking, motivations linked to care – that is, the motivations of women who look abroad to find a way of managing care responsibilities and improving the situation of their families – should be recognized. There is a "dark side" that comes with these motivations. First, women who feel they have no other choice than to look for opportunities abroad suffer abuse, exploitation, violence, and harmful health effects. The long-term consequences are often difficult to avoid as, when and if these women return home, they do not receive adequate care and support to enable them to reintegrate into society. Second, falling victim to sex trafficking further hampers the ability of women, who were motivated by caring responsibilities, to give and receive care. Indeed, migrating and falling victim to sex trafficking can damage family connections, leading to alienation between family members, erosion of emotional and kinship ties, family break-ups, and a variety of negative consequences flowing from women's being absent from the lives of their children. Robinson (2008b, 4) is correct, therefore, in raising the critical question: "While women sex workers ... are attending to the needs of their clients, who 'cares' for those workers (and their immediate and extended families)?"

From the perspective of care ethics it becomes apparent how nation-states, such as Ukraine, create conditions that make sustaining care difficult if not impossible. It becomes obvious why economic and social policies must work to enable people to carry out care work and responsibilities: it is because care is a fundamental need and because the effects of not facilitating its delivery clearly transcend the private sphere of individual trafficked women and their immediate families. Both migration and sex trafficking deplete countries of their female population, contributing, for instance, to Ukraine's current demographic crisis. Mobility is difficult to combine with family development: it can and does decrease fertility rates (Detlev 2009). Children of migrant females lose out on the experiences of family socialization; they lack pedagogical guidance, emotional and spiritual support, often end up in the category of "problem children," and are at increased risk for criminality (Tolstokorova 2009). Damaged family connections can also lead to the neglect of and lack of safety for aged family members. The export of female labour also affects economic productivity and development at home. Finally, the costs of responding to the problem of sex trafficking are, in all sectors (but especially in the health, social services, and legal sectors), significant and include providing the types of supports and services needed to assist victims to return to their home countries.

In sum then, responses to sex trafficking cannot simply come in the form of "repressive" strategies that focus on how to stop migration or that create legal responses to and result in prosecution of traffickers. As the UNDP (2007b, 2) argues, "there have been many calls from governments, donors and NGOs to do prevention work from the empowerment perspective, focusing on those at high risk of becoming victims of trafficking." A key component of this type of empowerment work, however, should not only pay attention to addressing poverty in a unidimensional and traditional manner; rather, effective interventions should link the overall economic and social context to the genuine inability of caregivers both to care well and to be well cared for. They should also take into account that caregiving practices can be seen as a form of agency, even if the context in which women seek to provide care makes it difficult for them to take up these practices in an effective manner. Thus, the goal should be to address, with the direct input of these caregiving "survivors" (and within the available economic means and policy resources), care deficits, which so heavily influence processes of economic migration and the risks associated with sex trafficking.

Conclusion

Knowledge of the political, economic, and social contexts that enable trafficking are important but are often disconnected from considerations of the centrality of care in human lives and the implications of caring motivations for understanding migration and sex trafficking. Taking Ukraine as an example, the application of a care ethic reveals important information that is often hidden when these interrelated transnational problems are analyzed. It is not merely that economic and social policies in Ukraine have resulted in poverty, forcing people to look elsewhere for economic opportunities, it is also that, because there are no adequate social safety nets, these policies have also made it impossible for women, who are most often in caregiving roles vis-à-vis their immediate and extended families, to fulfill their caregiving responsibilities. Revealing this largely unexamined dynamic leads to another perspective on sex trafficking and its victims and survivors: they are often driven by caring motivations in the context of significant care deficits. Thus, one important response to the international problem of sex trafficking is to consider how governments, both in Ukraine and beyond, can better provide the enabling conditions for care. What is therefore needed is not public retrenchment but, rather, more state responsibility directed towards care (Hankivsky 2004). Seen from this analytic perspective, the need, practice, and related priorities of care are of great political and public significance.

9 A Feminist Democratic Ethics of Care and Global Care Workers
Citizenship and Responsibility

JOAN C. TRONTO

At present, care work is rapidly becoming a transnational commodity (Baldassar 2007; Chang 2000; Ehrenreich and Hochschild 2002; Garrett 2007; Hochschild 2005; Hondagneu-Sotelo 2001; Parreñas 2001a; Shachar 2006; Tastsoglou and Dobrowolsky 2003; Zontini 2004).[1] Both skilled and unskilled workers, a large proportion of whom are women, are leaving their homes in less developed countries to work in more developed states. The remittances that they send home have become a central part of the political economy of less developed states, and the work that they perform is increasingly vital to the more developed states (High-Level Dialogue on International Migration and Development of the General Assembly of the United Nations 2006; Vila 2004). Thus, this pattern of transnational care commodification is likely to intensify.[2]

The transnational commodification of care is different from other forms of commodification in the global political economy because direct care work — the work required to prepare all humans to live each day, including care for the bodily needs of the infirm, frail, and young as well as of the adults who are healthy and the spaces in which they live — is not really a commodity. If a commodity is something for which one can receive money in exchange, then in some sense care work is a commodity. However, while people can be paid for their "work," measured by time spent, the measure of care resists being turned into just another good or service to be sold on the market. Given its often physical and psychic intimacy, good care grows out of the trust that develops among those giving and receiving care. That caring for an infant involves such trust might be obvious, but for people to give a cleaning person a key to their house also involves a high level of trust. Thus, care creates a *relationship* among the parties caring and being cared for: this relationship is not a "thing."

The question that I address in this chapter is whether a feminist democratic ethics of care can tell us anything different or special about the place of care in the global political economy. We might answer this question in the negative; that is, we might say that an ethics of care is about empathy, or that it privileges care relationships only among family members or members of the same community, or that it only concerns dyadic relationships of care. Or we might deny that there is anything distinctive about the care workers who cross national borders seeking work. After all, domestic workers are analogous to agricultural workers; doctors and pharmacists are analogous to highly skilled IT workers. But as soon as we are attentive to the nature of care, and to the requirements of a *feminist democratic* ethics of care, then we recognize the ethical seriousness of care work within whatever else we might want to discuss in the global political economy. This is so because care work, by its nature, is relational and entails responsibilities among actors in these relationships. Because these relationships are both structured by, made possible through, and shaped by their political, social, and economic contexts, a thorough accounting of these relationships requires a *political* process that is as broad as are the relationships themselves.

Since no institutions yet exist on the global level that function to allocate overall social and political responsibility, the politics of allocating responsibility must still be largely contained within the nation-state. Allocating care responsibilities, though, is not the same as distributing goods.[3] As a result, a feminist democratic ethics of care provides a more thoughtful and useful account of both the problems of and the solutions to the transnational commodification of care than do more standard theories of justice.

A Feminist Democratic Ethics of Care

What is a feminist democratic ethics of care? How does it differ from standard accounts of justice? Let me describe a feminist democratic ethics of care along the dimensions of its ontological, epistemological, ethical, and political contours.

Ontologically, as many scholars (such as Koggel 1998, 2006a, 2006b; Robinson 1999, 2008a; Robinson 2007; Groenhout 2004 inter alia) argue, a feminist ethics of care starts from a unique account of human nature. First, from the standpoint of a feminist ethics of care, individuals are conceived of as being *in relationships*. While individual liberty can still matter, it makes little sense to think of individuals as if they were Robinson Crusoe, all alone, making decisions. Instead, all individuals constantly work in, through, or away from relationships with others. Those others are in differing states of providing care for and needing care from them. Second, all humans are vulnerable and fragile. While it is true that some are more vulnerable than others, all humans are extremely vulnerable at some points in their lives, especially when they are young, elderly, or ill. Human life is fragile, and all of us are constantly vulnerable to changes in our bodily conditions that may require that we rely on others for care and support. Third, all humans are at once both recipients and givers of care. While the typical images of care indicate that those who are able-bodied and adult give care to children, the elderly, and the infirm, it is also the case that all able-bodied adults receive care from others, and from themselves, every day. And it is also the case that, except for very few people in states that approach catatonia, all humans engage in caring behaviour towards those around them. Children as young as ten months old imitate the activity of feeding; they open their mouths as they try to feed their caregiver (Bråten 2003). Children describe their activities as caring for parents (Mullin 2005). People are both givers and receivers of care all the time.

Epistemologically, feminist democratic care ethics differ from many other accounts of care ethics in that it relies upon an *expressive-collaborative*, rather than upon a theoretical-juridical, conception of morality. Margaret Urban Walker (1998, 2007) distinguishes these two kinds of approaches to metaethics. To Walker, the theoretical-juridical model allows philosophers to engage in discussions at a level of abstraction that grows out of a failure to recognize the distinctive location of philosophical discussion: "It also shields from view the historical, cultural, and social location of the moral philosopher, and that of moral philosophy itself as a practice of intellectual and social authority" (35). The usual basis for such claims is that moral philosophers have grounded their arguments in carefully honed philosophical standards of logic and reason. But, asks Walker, why do these standards bear special status in making moral argument? Why are moral philosophers exempt from the bias that they might attribute to all others? In contrast to this kind of argument, then, Walker suggests that a more appropriate way to understand ethics is to see them as an outcome of an expressive-collaborative process in which various moral actors come to an agreement about an acceptable set of moral standards. Expressive-collaborative morality thus makes no claim to being beyond time or place; rather, it "looks at moral life as a continuing negotiation *among* people" (60, emphasis in original). As Lorraine Code (2002, 160) elaborates: "Beginning and ending in practices of responsibility, both epistemic and moral, this model shifts attention to questions about how moral agents, singly and cooperatively, *express* their sense of self, situation, community, and agency in the responsibilities they discover and/or claim as theirs. Expressing and claiming are not impersonal processes but the actions of specifically identified, located deliberators, trying to work out how to live well in the circumstances in which they find themselves; starting not from an unstructured, uncontaminated 'original position' but from the possibilities and constraints consequent upon the hand they have been dealt." This approach "displaces formulaic deduction from theoretical principles with negotiated understandings; and displaces legislation from first principles or categorical imperatives with cooperative engagement in producing habitable communities, environments, and ways of life" (ibid.).

Ethically, a feminist democratic ethics of care draws upon several sets of moral qualities as key. They grow out of the complex processes of care itself. In *Moral Boundaries* (Tronto 1993), I identify four moral qualities that align with the four phases of care that Berenice Fisher and I identified in 1990. They are:

1 Caring about. At this first phase of care, someone or some group notices unmet caring needs. It calls for the moral quality of *attentiveness*, of a suspension of one's self interest, and a capacity, genuinely, to look from the perspective of the one in need. (In fact, we might also be attentive or inattentive to our own needs.)
2 Caring for. Once needs are identified, someone or some group has to take *responsibility*, its key moral quality, to make certain that these are met.
3 Caregiving. Assuming responsibility is not yet the same as doing the actual work of care, doing such work is the third phase of caring and requires the moral quality of *competence*. To be competent to care, given one's caring responsibilities, is not simply a technical issue, but a moral one.
4 Care receiving. Once care work is done, there will be a response from the person, thing, group, animal or plant, or environment that has been cared for. Observing that response, and making judgments about it (e.g., was the care given sufficient? successful? complete?) requires the moral quality of *responsiveness*.

Selma Sevenhuijsen (1998), reflecting on such practices, adds a more substantive set of concerns that distinguish care; they include making caring for physical vulnerabilities and dependency a priority and making a commitment to trust and respect. Although Sevenhuijsen published her book before Walker published *Moral Understandings,* she describes the moral qualities necessary for the *process* of what Walker identifies as the *substantive* significance of her metaethical position in calling her view an "ethics of responsibility." As Walker (1998, 4) puts it: "An "ethics of responsibility as a normative moral view would try to put people and responsibilities in the right places with respect to each other." Thus, the qualities identified by Sevenhuijsen help to identify the critical moral qualities that make it possible for people to take collective responsibility and to engage in the kinds of affixing of responsibility that Walker sees as fulfilling this metaethical need.[4] They are the moral dispositions and practices that make it possible to engage in the *processes* that will fix responsibility for care in society.

Politically, it is important to note that the kinds of discussions that Walker and Code envision informing an expressive collaborative morality, the kind of "judging with care" that Sevenhuijsen endorses, can only occur in a society in which real people have an opportunity to express themselves and to be heard by others. Only a democratic political order can enable this. In any other political order, even one that is "liberal" but not democratic, there is a claim of authority made on the part of some to trump the exchange of views in which all are able to participate.[5]

Caring democracy thus requires a commitment to genuine equality of power and voice, and the capacity for a meaningful democratic discussion of the nature of responsibility in society. However, often in contemporary discussions of democratic theory, such ends as equal power are simply posited, without the theorist's providing an account of how society can arrive at a place of greater equality. Political theorists usually seek procedural rather than substantive ways to address such challenges. Indeed, one of the major ways in which contemporary democratic theory is framed – deliberation versus "agonism" – is mainly about a difference in the nature of democratic dispute. Within each camp, then, there are further discussions of procedure but little engagement between (or within) these approaches about the substance of democratic discussion. What a democratic ethics of care requires, on the contrary, is a substantive focus on the allocation of responsibilities that includes all of the parties in the discussion. Thus, *democratic politics should centre on assigning responsibility for care.* The task of a democratic politics involves affixing responsibility, and, as we come to recognize the centrality of care for living a decent human life, the task of democratic politics needs to be much more fully focused upon care responsibilities: their nature, their allocation, and their fulfilment.

Fully to fill in the details of this last claim goes beyond the scope of this chapter, but let me provide a sketch of what a democratic politics of care, understood as fixing responsibility, requires. First, it requires that we specify "who" will participate in the process of making decisions. As political scientists have long noticed, who "sits at the table" to make decisions can have as large an effect on the outcome as can what the people who sit at the table do. The question of who gets to decide is a critical one.

Imagine a whole series of tables set up in a large room. At each table are the people who will make judgments about how to put people and responsibilities in relationship to each other. Let's call these the responsibility-setting games,[6] or circles of responsibility. Obviously, people will be able to affect the outcome of a responsibility-setting if they are able to *exclude* others from that process. Imagine a game about racial injustice in which one race is excluded from the process of setting responsibility.[7] Exclusion is one effective way of controlling the outcomes of a political process. Democratic theorists have long realized how important it is that, in order to create genuinely democratic outcomes games, everyone be included in processes such as responsibility-setting. Usually, the more powerful are able to exclude the less powerful: this is one of the things that it means to be more powerful.

But exclusion is not the only way to rig the outcome of a circle of responsibility. Another way is to *absent* oneself or one's group from the "people" whose roles are under discussion in the responsibility-setting game. If individuals or groups in society are granted a "pass" with regard to being assigned responsibility, then they are also effectively able to exercise power over the outcome by virtue of being able to absolve themselves of responsibility. I have previously labelled this kind of behaviour "privileged irresponsibility." Thus, when it comes to dividing up the responsibilities for managing a household, the traditional breadwinner model allows the head of the household (usually the husband in this traditional model) a "pass" from most daily domestic duties because he has already brought home the money that organizes the household (Weinbaum and Bridges 1979). But it is important to see this mechanism both from a moral perspective (as a way of shirking responsibility by claiming that one's own responsibilities lie in some other area) and from a political perspective (as a kind of power through which one is able to force others to accept responsibilities – perhaps even too many responsibilities – without having actually to make the case for one's own exclusion from the discussion).

Part of the obscurity of our current world and our inability to have honest political discussions about matters of great importance, then, has to do with our inability to make judgments about who is responsible. To some extent, such irresponsibility rests upon what Mills (1997) calls "epistemological ignorance" – our unwillingness to know anything about the lives of those who are dominated through structures such as racism (see also Pateman and Mills 2007). By controlling the "we," some are able to affect the apportioning of responsibility without really owning up to the responsibility of setting these conditions. Such exclusions and absences are thus vitally important in shaping how political discussions go forward.

What people will decide when they come together to allocate responsibility is another key issue. This matter is greatly complicated, of course, by the fact that "the table" at which they will sit always has a context. There is a history among these people, and past decisions and judgments shape what can be decided now. One never begins to think about responsibility with a clean slate.[8]

The matter is also complicated because we can think of responsibility in distinctive ways. One way to think of responsibility is to see it as "backward looking," as assigning blame for past judgments and actions. Usually, legal forms of assigning responsibility are "backward looking" in this way. This form of backward-looking responsibility has not received much of an endorsement from feminist writers. As Heidi Grasswick (2003, 92) observes, "many feminists have been uncomfortable with the judgmental language of responsibility that follows when praise and blame are taken to be its primary features." Indeed, she continues, "these concerns stem from a common view among these feminists that the language of responsibility, particularly when it is focused on praise and blame, reflects a preoccupation with purity" (93). Other feminist scholars also argue that "backward-looking" conceptions of responsibility are inappropriate tools for feminist analysis because feminists instead need an account of responsibility that helps direct future research (Card 2002; Young 2006).

In contrast, then, feminist scholars have begun to develop a model of responsibility that is forward-looking and that accounts for how to make change. For example, Iris Young (2006) writes about structural injustices and the social connection model of responsibility. Young's account of responsibility brings back a key element of the ontological starting point of care: that humans are involved in relationships, that the lines of these relationships can be traced, and that groups can then raise questions of responsibility. This is so even if efforts are made to disguise or to diminish responsibility (Pettit 2007).

On some level, then, the process of allocating responsibility is at the heart of the political practices of care. The political "care work" also requires that those accountable for the allocation of care responsibilities throughout society are attentive to whether or not those processes of care function. This can be done through a variety of means, but the best will require the participation of actual care workers and receivers in providing responses about how well caring needs are being met.

Questions about allocation of care responsibilities do not follow the traditional division of "left" and "right" in predictable ways (Sevenhuijsen 2000). Such a reallocation does require, however, that we rethink public and private duties and separations, whether needs can be defined collectively or individually, and whether people can be treated individually at the same time that they are treated equally.

What distinguishes a feminist democratic ethics of care from Margaret Walker's more general "ethics of responsibility" should now also be clear: a care ethics provides a substantive basis for applying the ethics of responsibility. It directs our attention to certain aspects of life in order to determine responsibilities. Some forms of responsibility can appear to be contractual, but, for an ethics of care, one needs always to go beyond simple agreements to look more closely at the power allocation in exchanges about responsibility. One also needs to focus upon relationships among people, and not simply upon isolated individuals, in making decisions about care.

While this assimilation of responsibility and responsibility to care may have begun to sound like a problem of distributive justice, and to some extent it is, we need to recall that politics is about power not only in the distributive sense but also in the sense of the creation or assumption of the collective capacity to act. Responsibility, Thomas Haskell reminds us, is a term that only entered the English language at the end of the eighteenth century. It requires that we see ourselves as capable of acting and as somehow implicated, causally, in the situation to be addressed (Haskell 1998). It is never, then, simply a matter of distribution. Furthermore, if "ought implies can," Haskell observes, then what follows is a very complicated understanding of what is necessary and what is transformable in human life and, hence, what constitute the limits of responsibility. How should we think, then, about the converse: to what extent does "can imply ought?" Haskell glosses Williams' discussion of slavery in the ancient world and observes that, since ancient writers simply assumed that slavery was necessary, they did not imagine it could be immoral. Haskell then asks, "How do 'necessary evils' such as slavery come to seem remediable, thus shrinking the domain of necessity and expanding the realm within which the imperatives of responsibility can operate?" (297).[9] From this standpoint – of what is beyond the scope of responsibility and what is within our power to change – Nancy Fraser's (1989b) concern about the "politics of needs interpretation" assumes a new salience. For if we are unwilling to question the necessity behind a set of practices, then we will not see ourselves as responsible for them.

In a democratic society, we might presume to say that everyone in the society should be around the table making decisions about the allocation of responsibilities. But, with limited time and resources, not everyone will be involved in every decision about allocating responsibility. One way to think about a society's political values, in the broadest possible terms, is to ask the question, what are the primary decisions that have been made about the allocation of responsibility? For example, if a society leaves questions about how much and what kind of education children should receive to their parents, then one allocation of a basic responsibility has been made about who sits at the table and makes judgments about the child's education. Whether this is a wise decision never reoccurs on the political agenda because the prior allocation to a very narrow circle of responsibility has already occurred. On the other end of this spectrum, allocations of responsibility also operate on a global level. If democracy should be a global value, the artificial limit of national sovereignty seems an unsatisfying answer to the question of whom to seat within the circles of responsibility that concern the safety and flourishing of people around the world (Goodhart 2005).

When we incorporate our concern about responsibility, we now see the main problems inherent in care – the problems of paternalism and parochialism (Tronto 1993) – in a new light. Both can now be understood as distortions of the kinds of responsibilities that people should appropriately assume. For paternalists, the problem is that they claim too much authority in the allocation of responsibility for themselves. Parochialism is a problem in which we set the boundaries of our responsibility too narrowly. In both of these cases, what will help us to better understand the moral problems that we face is to think about them in concrete terms: who is involved in making decisions, how are they involved, who have they excluded, and who is exercising various forms of privileged irresponsibility?

To review, a feminist democratic ethics of care requires that we reconceive democratic politics as the allocation of social and individual responsibilities, that we ensure the adequacy of the democratic process by making certain that people neither absent themselves nor exclude others from this process. The democratic process itself is no guarantee that members of a political community will arrive at the correct decision; however, including all in allocating responsibilities might make it less likely that some potential changes are hidden behind the claim of necessity, and it would make it less likely that paternalistic or parochial ideas would prevail without challenge. In the next section of this chapter, I compare how standard political theories of justice and a feminist democratic ethics of care differ in the ways that they understand the moral dimensions of transnational commodified care.

Evaluating the Moral Issues in Transnational Commodified Care: The Limits of the Justice Approach

From the start, it is clear that an ethics of care-based understanding of human nature, epistemology, morality, and politics differs from the understanding shaped in more traditional justice approaches to ethical questions. These different starting assumptions also affect how we assess moral issues within particular situations. In order to illustrate this point with reference to the global economy, let us consider the condition of care workers who are working transnationally.[10]

Within Anglo-American philosophy, the situation of care workers who have crossed borders has primarily been treated as a special case of more general concerns about immigration. They are seen as a group Joe Carens refers to as "irregular migrants" (Miller 2008a, 2008b; Carens 2008a, 2008b). Standard immigration arguments presume that, precisely because such migrants have often left members of their family behind (Ehrenreich and Hochschild 2002), they deserve *less* consideration than do other migrants as they are less likely to become permanent members of their new society. For Miller (2008a), the ambivalence of their commitment makes irregular migrants less committed to the contractual commitment to join the new society, and they therefore are not entitled to "citizenship rights." As for Carens (2008a), while he recognizes the dangers of exploitation in such arrangements, he is unwilling to condemn the Canadian live-in domestic program because, in the end, it may help a few thousand people who otherwise would not have access to Canada. In this same article, Carens challenges the position of Daniel A. Bell (2001), who defends the exploitative treatment of domestic workers in Singapore because, after all, they are still better off as domestics in Singapore than they were at home in, for example, Sri Lanka. Carens, in response to Bell, argues that the global political economic context of how maids end up doing such work matters.[11] Yet, surprisingly, he does not bring this same analysis to bear on the situation in Canada.

This problem reveals one of the issues involved in thinking about the morality of transnational commodified care from a perspective in which only one side of the situation is engaged, as opposed to the requirement set by Walker for "expressive collaborative" moral reasoning, in which "others" would have to be included in this discussion. The outcome, one might assume, would be different were they included.

As if to correct for the one-sidedness of these discussions, several feminist thinkers approach this question differently within the framework of traditional theories of justice. They draw upon the Kantian notion of "right to hospitality." In one of the rare cases in which thinkers have actually tried to think about justice from the standpoint of the particular kind of women care workers who are engaged in care transnationally, Wendy Sarvasy and Patrizia Longo argue that guest workers should be understood as world citizens and thus accorded the right of hospitality described by Immanuel Kant. Kant argues that, because "all nations are *originally* members of a community of the land," we all remain members not of "a legal community of possession" but of "a community of reciprocal action *(commercium)* in which members have "constant relations with all the others" (Sarvasy and Longo 2004, 396-97.) Sarvasy and Longo's argument is all the more appealing since, from the original Kantian standpoint, it is not clear whether the workers that they discuss would actually count as citizens. Kant's account of hospitality is directed at the peoples in the rest of the world, who, he thought, should be hospitable to European explorers.

In drawing a parallel between the household and the state, though, Kant inadvertently reveals the problem of basing rights on hospitality. The problem is that it depends upon the "friendly agreement" by which strangers are made into members of the household.[12] Now, Sarvasy and Longo take this argument to suggest that the visitors have a *political* role to play in making themselves welcome. The problem with this approach is that it still leaves the guest workers with the burden of demonstrating that they *deserve* membership. Kant also suggests (as Sarvasy and Longo note) that people have an imperfect duty to be sociable; thus, perhaps, people are obliged to listen to the arguments of their guests, but the burden still remains on the outsiders to explain why they should be admitted. And then, who shall be the judge? The right to hospitality never de-centres the position of the original citizen as "the one who was here first" and never challenges the basically unequal footing upon which original citizens and guest workers stand. What will make people challenge their own ethical views? To ask that newcomers alone "make the case" for their inclusion imposes an unequal and unfair burden upon them.[13] Traditional theories of justice are thus limited in their ability to solve the problems of transnational care commodification. At this point, a feminist democratic ethics of care offers more insight.

The Moral Problems of Transnational Commodification: The Advantages of a Feminist Democratic Ethics of Care

Let us now turn to the moral problems of the commodification of transnational care. Most of the discussions of injustice focus on distributive questions. Hence, Arlie Hochschild (2005, 13) describes the neglect of children of women who have migrated to care for the children of others as a question of distribution, but it gains its force from drawing upon a moral sensibility about the relationships of mothers and children: "Faced with these facts, one senses some sort of injustice at work, linking the emotional deprivation of these children with the surfeit of affection their First World counterparts enjoy."

The argument that I make about the nature of a feminist democratic ethics of care suggests a different language and logic by which to describe the moral question at issue here. Rather than using a language of *distribution,* which brings with it the notion that care is something that can be distributed, let us take seriously the idea that care is about relationships and that any democratic procedure within a state should recognize its transnational effects. John Stuart Mill (1998 [1859], 518) writes: "the true virtue of human beings is fitness to live together as equals." As Mill observes, the capacity to live together as equals requires a very specific kind of moral training, one in which no person is made to feel superior to others. From this perspective, the other harm brought about by transnational care commodification becomes clear: it violates this Millian possibility of equality.

Transnational care commodification is undemocratic because when immigrants are care workers, they become marked, as the anthropologists put it, with the stigma of care work. They are viewed as part of a feminized, multicultural workforce. They are distinctive because they are marked by a brutalized or privatized form of work.[14] They are different people in different regions and historical eras, but they are clearly designated as appropriate to do servile work and are marked by race, colour, religion, creed, accent, national origin, and so forth. In her volume *Sister/Outsider* Audre Lorde

(1984, 126) recounts: "I wheel my two-year-old daughter in a shopping cart through a supermarket in Eastchester in 1967, and a little white girl riding past in her mother's cart calls out excitedly, 'Oh look, Mommy, a baby maid!'" American culture often situates the multicultural person in the place of a servant whose role is to placate the concerns of white Americans who increasingly rely on such support (Wong 1994).

Yet, the harm of such marking is multifaceted. In the first place, it signals that marked people are better suited for care work and, thus, are not equals. This is a serious danger in a democratic society. Barbara Ehrenreich (2000, 70) observes that this has especially bad effects on children who learn that they do not need to learn to clean up after themselves:

> To be cleaned up after is to achieve a certain magical weightlessness and immateriality. Almost everyone complains about violent video games, but paid housecleaning has the same consequence-abolishing effect: you blast the villain into a mist of blood droplets and move right along; you drop the socks knowing they will eventually levitate, laundered and folded, back to their normal dwelling place. The result is a kind of virtual existence, in which the trail of litter that follows you seems to evaporate all by itself ... A servant economy breeds callousness and solipsism in the served, and it does so all the more effectively when the service is performed close up and routinely in the place where they live and reproduce.

One of the elements of the harm that Ehrenreich stresses is that it is exacerbated by being privatized and carried out in the household. As I argue elsewhere (Tronto 2002), I also believe that the moral dimensions of the exploitation of workers are worse in the household than elsewhere. This is so because household work is often not viewed as work at all, and household workers who do care work produce more intimate relationships than are produced in other kinds of work environments.

But a second harmful form of inequality is that, often, the needs of such individuals are taken to be different from the needs of the mainstream population. In many cases in which the values of multicultural groups have been juxtaposed to the views of mainstream groups in society, the courts seem to be willing to argue that, in such communities, the needs of people are different. Not only are they different, but they are lesser. Hence, in *Yoder*, the Supreme Court of the United States was willing to find that children from Amish communities do not need as much education as do other children. From such kinds of analyses, it will never be possible to arrive at a position of equality for individuals. From the standpoint of responsibility, it is easy to see that, on the one hand, such inequality would work to justify excluding servile people from a role in determining the allocation of public responsibility, and that, on the other hand, the powerful might absent themselves from the tasks of responsibility on the grounds that such concerns (i.e., those relating to the servile) are beneath them. In this way, the patterns of subordination continue.

Solving the Problems

If, as I suggest here, we need to think about care as a basic problem in allocating responsibilities in democratic societies, then the solution to the problems become clear: nations must extend citizenship to all those who are involved in substantive relations of care with citizens (Tronto 2005).

This proposal is congruent with an ethics of care and responsibility that requires all parties to be engaged in the setting of public and private responsibilities for care (and, by extension, in determining those boundaries). Only by making care workers participants in the discussion can we be somewhat assured that marking them as care workers will not create a lesser status for them. There are other implications of this view. Since the care work of transnational care workers often stretches beyond national limits, all of the care relations in which a care worker is involved should make her or him eligible for citizenship *by virtue of her/his care relationship with those who are engaged in caring relations with citizens*. This broadening of citizenship permits us to rethink the nature of states, of security (Robinson 2008a), and of the role of citizens.

We can imagine many objections to this kind of approach. First, in the recent past, following T.H. Marshall, what has qualified citizens for membership is their economic contribution to the productive forces of society. Caring for people is not a contribution on the same order. It equates care in private life with a public good. This objection is easily answered: care in private life *is* a public good (Folbre 1994, 2001). Every human society depends upon the production of citizens through their birth and child rearing. Every worker must be "reproduced" in order to survive and to return to work the next day (Weinbaum and Bridges 1979). Furthermore, when Marshall equates productive work with a contribution to citizenship, he has already blurred the line between public and private contributions. Most workers work for private firms whose profit is not a social benefit. While both the firms and the individual workers are taxed, and through such taxes make a public contribution, the primary beneficiary of the work of citizens is not the state or "the economy" but the firms whose profits flow from the workers' efforts. Why should this kind of private contribution count as a public good when the private contribution of caring for people does not?[15]

Second, expanding the state's realm of concern beyond its physical territory to include people who may not live in the territory and whose connection to it might be only through a single individual weakens that state's ability to protect itself. How can the state be expected to protect its "care chain" citizens who are scattered about the globe? And suppose some of these far-flung citizens decide to exercise their rights (e.g., by voting from distant locations and with little connection to local issues)?

While this objection exacerbates the vulnerability of the state, it is already a fact that no state can really guarantee the safety of its citizens. States are vulnerable not only within their own territories but also elsewhere in the world. States are already vulnerable to physical violence both at home and abroad. Were states to recognize this vulnerability, they might make better decisions in an increasingly connected international order. The greater distance of some citizens from their "home" state is not a strong argument against this approach. Even now, states are vulnerable to citizen who are disengaged from political life and to citizens who exercise their citizenship rights without much attentiveness and responsibility (Macedo and al. 2005). But these problems are not unique to care-chain citizens. Including such citizens, furthermore, might bring with it additional and diverse perspectives that can prove beneficial to states.

Third, some might object that transnational care workers have not done enough to earn their citizenship. In order to take this objection seriously, though, we need to ask whether the accident of birth in a particular nation-state should be "enough" to earn citizenship? The family members of transnational care workers do end up making sacrifices for the absent "commodity" of the transnational carer. Why should this contribution not suffice as grounds for citizenship?

Recognizing "in-country" variations in citizens who are in relationships with transnational care workers will also allow for a more robust understanding of cultural diversity within subgroups in any given society. As Werbner (2005) argues, paradoxically, a new multicultural community will often need to reinforce its own customs, ways of life, and so on before it can become fully integrated into a new culture. Werbner thus recognizes the importance of historical sensitivity in making judgments about newcomers. In a parallel way, it is important to make concessions about how caregiving practices work in some communities in order to make judgments about how members of those communities should be evaluated and integrated into society as a whole. For example, among some migrant groups, older children may have to share child-care responsibilities with parents. If such caregiving keeps boys and girls from participating in school events, they may appear less engaged when college admissions officers look at their records. They may lose out on future opportunities because they have taken on caregiving roles that were necessary or expected in their own community. In order for university officials to be just, then, they need to consider something more than a standard measure of "participation" that would apply to everyone.

Conclusion

The feminist democratic ethics of care brings a different perspective to the ethical questions of the global political economy than do the perspectives that currently dominate its discussion in political theory. Escaping from the fruitless antinomies of universalism/particularism, justice/democracy, and liberalism/communitarianism, the feminist democratic ethics of care posits that the questions of actual relationships, and the attendant responsibilities that they bring, provide a more coherent and action-oriented way to consider the problems of justice raised in the global political economy.

Conclusion
Integrating the Ethics and Social Politics of Care

RIANNE MAHON AND FIONA ROBINSON

The chapters in this book clearly demonstrate that an ethics of care cannot be separated from social politics and vice versa. On the contrary, an ethics of care that is political and critical must be grounded in the concrete activities of real people and the webs of social relations that connect them. At the same time, feminist students of social policy critically interrogate the gendered assumptions that underlie current care policies and practices. The conclusion is that new thinking is required – thinking that can disturb and challenge existing dichotomies and the compartmentalization of spheres of life, especially as these illuminate the contemporary processes of the commodification and transnationalization of care.

The commodification and transnationalization of care are taking place in a global context deeply marked by the ecological dominance of neoliberal ideas and practices as well as changing gender relations. In the global North, women's rising labour force participation rates and demographic changes (population aging, declining fertility) are giving rise to demands on fiscally restrained states to deal with the deepening care deficit. Our two chapters on Japan (Onuki; Tsuji) as well as Peng's analysis of recent developments in Korea nicely illustrate the way in which these contradictory pressures fuel the processes of commodification and transnationalization in the child- and elder-care sectors, while Gabriel's study of nurse migrants to Canada shows how these processes are also integral to health-care restructuring. In the global South, IMF-sponsored structural adjustment policies prompt states to encourage the out-migration of care workers as they become increasingly reliant on the flow of remittances. The Philippine government has been particularly active in this regard (Parreñas 2000); but is by no means alone.

This leads to the second point: commodification and transnationalization are not spontaneous, market-generated processes. To be sure, the emergence and expansion of for-profit providers, operating at the transnational as well as at national and local scales, plays its part (Williams, this volume), as do a welter of overseas recruitment and placement agencies, operating alongside NGOs and informal networks (Yeates 2004b). And, as Onuki and Hankivsky stress, it is important to recognize the agency of migrant caregivers themselves – in choosing to migrate as well as in contesting the terms of their admission. Yet states have not lost their importance. Their social and immigration policies and practices play a critical role. The lack of attention to the role of the state in the "global care-chain literature" perhaps reflects the latter's American origins. As Williams argues, "the global care chain emerged from research on the United States as the receiving country and, as such, identifies lack of public care provision in shaping the demand for child and elder care. In Europe, however, it is not simply the absence of the state provision in care that shapes the demand for ... care and the supply of migrant care but, rather, the restructured nature of the state support that is available" (this volume, 22). Elsewhere, Williams and her colleagues document how recent policy developments – in the form of cash provision, tax credits, and tax breaks as well as direct payments to care-receivers – in many Western European countries have helped to boost markets for child and elder care (Lister et al. 2007). Similarly, Onuki and Tsuji show the active role played by the Japanese state in creating a functioning care market through recent social and immigration policy initiatives. Gabriel details the ways in which Canadian immigration policy structures the inflow of nurses while, on the supply side, Hankivsky highlights the importance of the adverse impact of structural adjustment on women's ability to care for their families at home.

States may continue to play a critical role in the commodification of care and the construction of global care chains, but they do not do so in isolation. As Williams reminds us, we also need to take into account the transnational flow of care discourses and policies. We have already referred to the importance of structural adjustment policies promoted by the IMF and the World Bank for the global South and the countries of the former Soviet Bloc. For the global North, the OECD operates as a purveyor of neoliberal policy prescriptions (Mahon and McBride 2008). In this volume, Mahon argues that both the OECD and the World Bank have gone beyond what might be called the "brute neoliberalism" of the 1980s to embrace a social investment paradigm. While the Bank's version thereof is perhaps best considered "neoliberalism plus," the OECD's interpretation is more open to policies designed to promote gender equality.

How do we unravel the impact of these international organizations on domestic policy agendas? One strand of the literature emphasizes "policy learning," but the latter always involves a process of "translation," in which travelling ideas, like the social investment paradigm, "are combined with already existing institutional practices and, therefore, translated into local practice in varying degrees" (Campbell 2004, 80). The chapters by Peng and Tsuji provide nice examples of this process. As Peng shows, through the role played by transnational epistemic communities, the Korean governments of Kim Dae-jung and Roh Moo-hyun were exposed to the social investment paradigm and learned from social investment experiments elsewhere. At the same time, in contrast to New Labour's policies in Britain, which emphasized skills development and retraining, Korea's policies were designed to deal with demographic concerns (population aging, fertility decline) and the need to create service-sector employment. Tsuji's analysis goes one step further, bringing out the complex ways in which neoliberal, gender equality, and familialist discourses combined to shape the translation process.

More broadly, seen from the standpoint of a critical ethics of care, although the social investment paradigm may open up space for addressing care needs, it leaves undisturbed the familiar opposition between states and markets, individuals and communities. In her critique of Third Way discourse in Britain, Selma Sevenhuijsen argues that it remains marked by oppositions between the individual and society. By contrast, a feminist ethic of care begins by denying such oppositions between individuals and society. It provides an "alternative view on the creation of social ties compared to that of the building of bridges between individuals and society" (Sevenhuijsen 2000, 9). The social investment discourse also sidesteps "crucial issues of women's empowerment" and fails to challenge the subservience of care policies to economic development (Williams, this volume).

Moreover, the normative thrust behind the idea of "investing in children" remains explicitly tied to economic growth, heightened labour productivity, and securing "future sources of wealth" (Suh 2007, quoted in Peng, this volume). While some care ethicists argue that market values should not have priority in education, child care, and health care (Held 2002), others argue for a more nuanced analysis of the outdated rhetoric surrounding states, markets, and their relationship to care (Folbre and Nelson 2000). In a particularly compelling analysis, Susan J. Smith argues that the persistent divide among states that manage politics, markets that perform the economy, and caring communities whose work is anchored in the spaces of the home constitutes a "political geography in which the economic imperatives of competitive individualism ... have become detached from an intrinsically relational ethic of care." Such partitioning, she argues, has been "spectacularly successful in constraining the imagery of what states can and should do ... and [has] left the dispassionate workings of the market surprisingly intact" (Smith 2005, 1-2). In the meantime, however, as we work towards the formulation of a new, more creative political geography, it is important to recognize and address the harms caused by the ways in which welfare societies are seeking to reduce their social expenditure costs through the commodification of care (Williams).

While much has been written about the need to deconstruct the public/private dichotomy that has for so long relegated the values and practices of care to the household, less attention has been paid to other dichotomies that also serve to constrain innovative ethical and political thinking. For the ethics of care, perhaps the most crucial of these is the autonomy/dependence dichotomy. Some feminist critics of care ethics argue that an ethics of care valorizes women's dependence, thus leading to the reification of gender stereotypes. What this critique misses is the emphasis in most accounts of care ethics on interdependence and on the mutually constitutive nature of autonomy and dependence. From this perspective, interdependence is a defining feature of social life; it shapes and defines identity and influences well-being. Interdependence is neither a natural nor simply a private condition; rather, it is created by and mediated through social and political institutions. Vulnerability and dependence, moreover, are features of all human subjects as well as many social groups at some point in their existence; levels of vulnerability, and the implication of vulnerability are, in part, a reflection of existing power relations in the context of relationships. Thus, if women, and especially women of colour, appear to be less autonomous than men, it is in part due to the ways in which their dependence has been constructed through norms of race and gender and their relationship to caring labour.

In policy terms, the shift from the "male breadwinner" model to the "adult-earner family model" has given rise to the need for extrafamilial care and has put pressure on states to support this (Williams; Tsuji; Peng). Unless the prevailing dichotomous thinking is challenged, this move will be seen as the failure of individual families (including female-headed, single-parent families) to remain autonomous. What is required is a recognition and acceptance of the reality of vulnerability and dependence for all people at some times in their lives. This is not to say, however, that autonomy, and the associated norms of individual freedom and human rights, should not be valued; rather, as Williams (2000, 481) argues, the task is less one of arguing against autonomy as a liberal concept than one of redefining the concept of autonomy to fit with a notion of interdependence. The ethics of care recognizes that autonomy is neither naturally achieved nor necessarily sustainable in the long term. While rights to secure independence and a meaningful voice in politics are strategically and discursively important for individuals and groups, true autonomy for *all* can only be achieved and sustained in and through fostering societies that value interdependence and that acknowledge the vulnerability of all (ibid.).

The need to reconsider our conventional views of autonomy and dependence is also important at the state level in the international system. Recognition of the increasing dependence of the North on the South for the provision of care work challenges conventional understandings of the South as "dependent" on the North. When viewed through a critical care lens, what Sassen calls "counter-geographies" of globalization are revealed. Sassen's analysis uncovers the systemic connections between poor migrant women (often represented as a burden rather than as a resource) and significant sources for profit and government revenue enhancement. The lines of dependency, from this perspective, are striking: "I use the notion of feminization of survival to refer to the fact that households and whole communities are increasingly *dependent* on women for their survival. It is important to emphasize that governments too are *dependent* on their earnings as well as enterprises where profit making exists at the margins of the 'licit' economy" (Sassen 2002, 258 [emphasis added]). The aim of this line of argumentation is not simply to turn the autonomy/dependency dichotomy on its head; rather, it is to demonstrate that the nature and extent of dependence and interdependence in social, political, and economic life is constantly shifting and evolving, with different kinds of costs and benefits for different actors. Frameworks for social policy, and the ethics that support them, must revise their understandings of politics of dependence and autonomy if care concerns are to be adequately addressed.

A final dichotomy that can no longer be sustained in this context is the national/global divide. Key normative concepts in political philosophy, including citizenship, democracy, and distributive justice, can no longer be addressed simply at the level of the nation-state. From the perspective of care, however, the remedy to this is not simply to "globalize" these concerns from a universalist or cosmopolitan perspective. Nor does rethinking global justice using a care lens require simply adding more care options; rather, it requires reframing care through reference to the practices and ethics of interdependence, contextual sensitivity, responsiveness, and responsibility for the consequences of choice (Williams, this volume). Tronto's chapter in this volume advocates a feminist democratic ethics of care as an alternative to standard accounts of justice. While standard accounts focus on procedures for arriving at goals such as equality, a democratic ethics of care provides a substantive focus by centring upon *"assigning responsibility for care"* (Tronto, this volume). Crucially, Tronto points out that questions of responsibilities to care cannot simply be rolled into the framework of distributive justice; we need to recall, she argues, that "politics is about power not only in the distributive sense but also in the creation or assumption of the collective capacity to act" (Tronto, this volume, 169).

The increasing irrelevance of the national/global divide also pertains to the question of citizenship in the context of the transnational care economy. As many of the contributors to this volume point out, it may be useful to consider contemporary citizenship as multi-scalar – that is, to recognize multiple and overlapping citizenships and, significantly, to expand the scope of citizenship activities to include the practices and labour associated with care. That said, it is crucial to avoid the development of hierarchies of citizenship. One of the effects of transnational commodified care is the marking of certain people as being better suited for care and as having different, usually lesser, needs than others (Tronto, this volume). When care work and caring practices are recognized as valuable activities of citizenship, the idea of broadening citizenship to include those "involved in substantive relations of care with citizens" takes on a new relevance.

Notes and Acknowledgments

INTRODUCTION

1 Or "trilemma," as Iversen and Wren (1998) argue: "Baumol's disease (the productivity gap between services and goods-production referred to by Himmelweit) means that countries cannot simultaneously pursue full employment, income equality and fiscal balance. The liberal regimes have focused on full employment and fiscal balance at the expense of inequality; social democratic regimes, full employment and income equality at the expense of high government expenditures; conservative regimes, equality and fiscal restraint at the expense of (service) employment" (Esping-Andersen 1999).

2 There is also Nancy Fraser's (1997) important "thought experiment" in which she assesses the universal breadwinner, caregiver parity, and universal caregiver models for their impact on gender equality.

CHAPTER 1: TRANSNATIONAL ANALYSIS OF THE POLITICAL ECONOMY OF CARE

Two projects have stimulated this research. The first was funded by the European Community's Sixth Framework Programme (ref. MEIF-CT-2003-502369). Between July 2004 and April 2005, Anna Gavanas carried out interviews in London, Stockholm, and Madrid with a total of 102 migrant care workers and employers of such workers and agencies. I am grateful to Anna Gavanas for her interviews and translations. I am also grateful to the ESRC for funding the study titled *A Theoretical Synthesis of Gender, Migration and Care, and Welfare Regimes* (ref. ESRC 000-22-1514), which was undertaken as part of an ongoing research collaboration with scholars from Ireland, Germany, and the Netherlands studying migrant work in child care and elder care in Europe (in a project titled *Migration and Networks of Care*) under the Eurocores program, 2006-09.

1 Here Parreñas extends Sassen's analysis of the "international division of labour" as one of the key elements of globalization.
2 Yeates (2009, fig. 3.4, p. 6) identifies nineteen different types of agencies outside the state.
3 Although Asis (2006), cited by Kofman and Rhaguram (2007), finds that fathers played an important role.
4 Although some reports identify a merging of male and female behaviour in certain instances.
5 *ABC Sale Process*, http://www.childcare.com.au/.
6 Yeates (2009) also notes the importance of transnational religious care discourses in care chains.
7 See "Who Cares? Care Services for All Women and Men in Europe," http://www.womenlobby.org/.
8 The UN Convention on the Rights of Persons with Disabilities focuses on respect, autonomy, and independence; on freedom from discrimination; and on inclusion, participation, and equality.
9 From the World Bank Conference in Arusha Tanzania entitled "New Frontiers of Social Policy."
10 Nor about the impact of global neoliberal policies on women and their opportunities for and conditions of work (see Molyneux and Razavi 2006). These arguments about the contradictions in gender mainstreaming also apply to the European Union. See, for example, the special issue of *Social Politics* 12, 3 (2005), especially Daly.
11 There are, of course, exceptions, and there is not room here to account for the detailed critiques provided, for example, by Beneria (2003), Elson (2004), Hassim (2006), Katz (2001), Pearson (2004), Kabeer (1994), and Yeates (2004a). See also Robinson's (2006b) critique of Pogge.
12 This paragraph draws on Hankivsky (2004).

CHAPTER 2: MIGRATION AND GLOBALIZED CARE WORK

I am grateful to Leah Vosko for her astute comments on an earlier draft of this chapter.

1 Throughout this chapter, "skill" is recognized as a socially constructed category. See Gabriel (2004).
2 Following Blythe and Baumann (2009, 192), I use IEN "interchangeably with *migrant*. However, it is important to note that a minority of IENs are Canadians educated abroad and migrants who are educated in Canada are not IENs." Further, the IEN designation includes different nursing groups. For the most part, I focus on the case of registered nurses (RNs).
3 The arguments presented in this section draw directly on Gabriel (2008).
4 The federal government of Canada established this commission in 2001 to evaluate Canada's publicly funded health-care system and make policy recommendations to improve the system and its future sustainability. It was headed by Roy J. Romanow, QC. After extensive consultations, the commission tabled its final report, *Building on Values: The Future of Health Care in Canada* (http://www.hc-sc.ca/).

CHAPTER 3: THE GLOBAL MIGRATION OF CARE LABOUR

This chapter is a revised, updated, and shortened version of an article entitled "Care, Social (Re)production and Global Labour Migration: Japan's 'Special Gift' toward 'Innately Gifted' Filipino Workers," *New Political Economy* 14, 4 (2009): 489-516 (reprinted by permission of the publisher, Taylor and Francis Ltd., http://www.informaworld.com). I wish to thank the editors of this volume plus Stephen Gill, Natsue Okamura, Deepa Rajkumar, Adrienne Roberts, and Yuki Tsuji for their insightful criticisms and comments on previous versions of this chapter.

1 "What is considered socially acceptable for care work," as Kate Bezanson and Meg Luxton (2006, 3-4) point out, will vary in different times and spaces, but this chapter primarily focuses on "elder care" in Japan.
2 In August 2008, 205 Indonesian nurse and care-worker candidates entered Japan (*Mainichi Shimbun* 2008b). Further, Japan is currently discussing the possibility of receiving Thai care workers through the recently ratified EPA with Thailand (MOFA 2007a, 2011).
3 For the details, see Mori (1997) and Hanami and Kuwabara (1989).
4 This chapter is based on ethnographic research that I conducted from February to August 2007 in Japan and the Philippines, including interviews with students in Filipino caregiving schools, their graduates who were receiving training to work in Japan, licensed Filipino care helpers residing in Japan, state officials, business groups, and nongovernmental or nonprofit organizations.
5 Interview with a MHLW official, 8 June 2007. Emphasis by the author.
6 Suzuki (2007) and Yamazaki (2006) underline the gaps in meanings and qualifications between the Japanese *kaigo fukushishi* and Filipino caregivers.
7 Interview with a MHLW official, 8 June 2007. The MHLW claims that there are approximately 200,000 potential care workers who hold the certificates but currently are not practising their professions (*Mainichi Shimbun* 2008a).
8 Currently, about 1,100,000 workers are engaged in the caregiving sector; however, according to the MHLW, the rapid growth of the elderly will require 400,000 to 600,000 new workers in the next ten years (*Mainichi Shimbun* 2008a). The MHLW also estimates that, by 2030, the number of total labourers will drop by 10 million from its current level to 56 million, and one in every twenty will have to be employed in the caring industry in order to maintain the current level of care provision (Vij 2007, 172-73).
9 Interview with an AOTS official, 4 July 2007. The official said that the capacity of AOTS to handle six hundred care workers in two years is highly questionable and, more essentially, that teaching "foreign" students in the field of caregiving is new for the institutions.
10 The names of Filipino care workers/caregivers/care helpers and caregiving students whom I quote in this chapter are all pseudonyms.
11 Interview with Takahashi, 12 May 2007.
12 Interview with B-Dimayuga, 25 May 2007.
13 Interview with an official at the Japanese Embassy in the Philippines, 21 May 2007.
14 Interview with Takaki Kojima at IPS Tokyo Caregiving Academy, 12 June 2007). See also Tanaka (2007).

Notes to pages 70-107

15 Interview with Kojima, 12 June 2007.
16 I owe these ideas to Chiho Ogaya.
17 Interview with Junta Shinozawa, the advisor of LFCAJ, 23 June 2007. Information about LFCAJ is available at http://www.ja-phil.com/.
18 Interview with the representative of a Japanese nonprofit organization, 15 June 2007.

CHAPTER 4: TRANSNATIONALIZING (CHILD) CARE POLICY

An earlier version of this chapter was published as "After Neo-Liberalism? The OECD, the World Bank and the Child," in *Global Social Policy* 10, 2 (2009): 183-204.

1 Early childhood education and care (ECEC) refers to the integration of child care and early child education. Early child development (ECD) has a broader scope, including things like prenatal care and parental education as well as ECEC. I use ECEC to refer to the transnational discourse in general and ECD only when I turn to the World Bank's version.
2 See Naim (1999) for a summary of the core features of the Washington Consensus, which lies behind the structural adjustment policies of the IMF and the World Bank.
3 Interestingly, both publications link the World Bank's conversion to primary over tertiary education to the "dazzling success" of East Asian countries like Korea. While it is true that the latter did invest in basic education for all, it also invested in higher education. Moreover, the Bank continued to ignore the larger role played by the "developmental state," no doubt because the latter's very active intervention in the economy flew in the face of the structural adjustment it favoured.
4 See "Early Childhood Development," on the World Bank's website.
5 Recognizing that many women are involved in the informal economy, Beneria argues, inter alia, for increasing access to neighbourhood child care and giving children access to neighbourhood schools. This is, in fact, the practice in countries (like Sweden) that have eschewed workplace-based child care.

CHAPTER 5: SOCIAL INVESTMENT POLICY IN SOUTH KOREA

1 Prior to 2004, child-care support was available only to low-income families.
2 Most of these programs focus on job creation and training to prepare women to work in elder-care services.
3 Also interview with Lee Sook Jin, Korea Institute of Health and Social Affairs (KIHASA), 18 December 2007.
4 Haekwons are private educational institutions specializing in providing English, music, arts, sports, and so on to children who are three to five years old.
5 Interview with Seung-Ah Hong, fellow, Family Policy Research Centre, KWDI, 14 December 2007.
6 Interview with Seung-Ah Hong, 14 December 2007. Hong was also involved in the KWDI research on child care during the child-care policy reform process in 2005 and 2006.
7 Interview with Joo-Hyun Park, secretary general and chairman of the Operating Committee, the Presidential Committee on Aging Society and Population Policy, 17 December 2007.

CHAPTER 6: REIMAGINED INTIMATE RELATIONS

1 In 1994, the Liberal Democratic Party agreed with its coalition partners, the Social Democratic Party of Japan and the New Party Sakigake, that the government would promote gender equality in society. In 1999, the Basic Law for a Gender-Equal Society passed in the Diet, and the national machinery for gender equality was established.
2 The prices are officially determined by the MHLW. At the same time, these official prices of elder-care services affect the wages that care workers receive.
3 While the amount of cash allowance proposed by conservative politicians in the Liberal Democratic Party was extremely low, it did not cover either accident or pension insurance, both of which are covered under the German system. In sum, while, in Germany, "caring for the elderly is genuinely viewed as 'work' and the cash allowance as 'pay'" (Webb 2003, 49), a cash allowance in Japan is seen as a token payment expressing gratitude to women for providing care in the household.
4 However, it is necessary to examine the intention of business carefully as the deregulation of the labour market and the growth of flexible employment have been encouraged since the late 1990s.
5 Since the MHLW deregulated requirements for obtaining licences to establish childcare facilities, the number of private providers has been increasing and that of public providers has been decreasing.
6 According to an opinion poll, the ratio of respondents who answered "yes" to the question "Do you feel or expect child-raising to be pleasant more often than painful?" remains at 42.9 percent (Cabinet Office 2002b).
7 This alliance influenced public education reforms in the 2000s. Today, students are taught family values and child-rearing knowledge (Cabinet Office 2008a, 107).
8 According to degrees of familialism and defamilialism (Leitner 2003), Japanese child care may be categorized as "explicit familialism." On the other hand, although the LTCI was supposed to create "defamilialism" (i.e., no cash and a wide range of care services), the actual situation of Japanese elder care remains "implicit" or "explicit familialism" (i.e., no care provisions outside the family, with or without financial assistance for family caregiving). Japan institutionalized paid parental leave, and the ratio of children under three in formal care services is 15.2 percent (OECD 2007). The percentage of people over sixty-five receiving home help services remains about 10 percent (calculated by author based on information in MHLW 2005b).

CHAPTER 7: CARE ETHICS AND THE TRANSNATIONALIZATION OF CARE

Parts of this chapter are derived from Fiona Robinson, *The Ethics of Care: A Feminist Approach to Human Security* (Philadelphia: Temple University Press, 2011).

1 Porter cites Robinson (2001, 1999) as a "notable exception" to this.
2 The terms "critical moral ethnography," "moral understandings," and "social-moral systems" are taken from Walker (1999). Elsewhere, I elaborate in detail on Walker's epistemology and methodology as a framework for feminist normative IR theory. See Robinson (2006c).
3 On the relationship between care ethics, care work, and human security, see Robinson (2008b).

4 A notable exception is Kershaw, Pulkingham, and Fuller (2008).
5 The extent to which race is a useful concept for the analysis of trafficking in women is contested. Laura M. Agustin argues that the fastest-growing group of migrants comes from Eastern Europe and the former Soviet Union – women usually considered "white" and "almost" European. Thus, she says, although "exoticizing" may well be taking place, race is not a useful analytical concept at this time (Agustin 2003, 378).
6 Sassen (2002, 220 and 271) notes that the Philippine government, through the Philippines Overseas Employment Administration (PIEA), has played an important role in the emigration of Philippine women – as maids, nannies, nurses, and "brides" – from the Philippines to the United States, the Middle East, and Japan.

CHAPTER 8: THE DARK SIDE OF CARE
1 The percentage of women below the poverty line is roughly similar or only slightly higher than the percentage of men below the poverty line.
2 K. Cherepakha, 2009. Interview by author at headquarters of La Strada, Kyiv, Ukraine, 11 May.

CHAPTER 9: FEMINIST DEMOCRATIC ETHICS OF CARE AND GLOBAL CARE WORKERS
1 There is an ongoing scholarly discussion about what constitutes care work. Here the term is used very broadly. At a minimum, care work includes the direct caregiving to human bodies as well as to the cleaning and maintenance of the spaces in which humans live and work. More broadly, organizing such care is also caregiving; for example, workers at an agency that arranges migrant home-help workers is also part of this transnational commodification of care work. For a justification of expansive readings of the meaning of care and care work, see Tronto (1993, 2005).
2 Since the economic downturn of 2008-09, there are many reports that the number of migrant workers is in decline and that, as unemployment grows, migrants are treated with greater hostility (e.g., Bilefsky 2009). Nonetheless, the structural circumstances that create such migration have not changed, and we can expect, unless there are major policy changes, that such migration patterns will escalate with a global economic recovery.
3 This insight derives from the critique of distributive models of justice offered by Iris M. Young (1990).
4 Ruth Groenhout also recognizes, in a somewhat different manner, that the moral quality of responsibility is, in some ways, the most public quality of care. Groenhout (2004, 46-57) does not use the language of responsibility, but her description of "finitude and interdependence" as elements of care that determine "all those who are capable of responsible action" (46-47) is parallel.
5 For example, liberals often place confidence in an independent judiciary to interpret laws so that "the rule of law" and appropriate legal protections are in place. See, for example, Dworkin (2000) and Nussbaum (1987, 2004, 2007).
6 Peter French (1992) describes a different "Responsibility Barter Game." I am indebted to Walker (2007, 101) for this reference.

7 In *The Racial Contract*, Charles Mills (1997) writes about an old African-American saying: "when white people say 'justice,' they mean 'just us.'"
8 Two thinkers who, in very different contexts, make a similar point are: Margaret Walker (2006), who discusses justice after wrongdoing, and Naomi Klein (2007), who argues that applying the Friedmanesque wish for a "clean slate" is anti-humanistic.
9 See also Hochschild (2005).
10 The stituations of transnational care workers are not all the same, of course: those who have migrated and form part of the "brain drain" are different from those who form part of the "care drain." Space limitations prevent a more nuanced discussion of their different circumstances, but, despite profound differences in circumstance, some similar arguments about the context of their decisions to move, the difficulties that they face, and so forth, can be made. See, inter alia, Kofman (2004).
11 Carens (2008a, 441) writes, as a response to Bell: "Take the claim in the inevitability argument that the only alternative to legal guestworkers with limited rights is irregular migrants with no effective rights at all. Why do these irregular migrants come? ... If states respond to migration pressures by implicitly tolerating or even encouraging irregular migration, as many states have done, especially with respect to seasonal workers in agriculture, they can then hardly eschew responsibility for the irregular migrants on their territory."
12 Once "those who were there first" get to decide whether the newcomers are being good guests, we have returned to the kind of analysis, it seems, that Walzer (1983) made.
13 Seyla Benhabib (2004, 94) tries to carry this "right to hospitality" further. She believes that a dialogue will resolve the problem between "the immigrant and the members of the host state where the latter must be able to show with good grounds that are acceptable to each equally, why the former will not be granted membership" (quoting Payrow Shabani's [2007] discussion of Benhabib). But because Benhabib's (2004) dialogue remains highly formal, it is difficult to know whether it would better represent the genuine interests and concerns of the otherwise excluded "irregular migrants." Why would not a Walzerian assertion meet the formal requirements here? "I have a right here to determine membership, just as you had a right there, wherever you were born, to determine membership, and so we are equally empowered in this way." Benhabib's solution turns out to be no solution at all.
14 This pattern of marking is more severe for the least qualified care workers, but it also affects doctors and nurses. One in six British health-care workers reported being bullied, especially by immediate supervisors, but among ethnic minorities the number increased to three in ten (International Centre for Human Resources in Nursing 2008).
15 A different concern might be that "privacy" will be violated if people discuss their care roles in public. For a distinction that helps to explain how to preserve "privacy" while providing accountability, see Allen (2003).

References

Abbott, Pamela, and Claire Wallace. 2007. Talking about health and well-being in post-Soviet Ukraine and Russia. *Journal of Communist Studies and Transition Politics* 23, 2: 181-202.

Abu-Laban, Yasmeen, and Christina Gabriel. 2002. *Selling diversity: Immigration, multiculturalism, employment equity and globalization*. Peterborough, ON: Broadview Press.

Ackers, Louise, and Helen Stalford. 2004. *A community for children: Children, citizenship and internal migration in the EU*. Aldershot: Ashgate.

Action on Disability and Development. 2009. Disability facts. http://www.add.org.uk/.

Adamson, Peter. 2008. *The child care transition: A league table of early childhood education and care in economically advanced countries*. UNICEF Innocenti Research Centre, Report Card 8. http://www.unicef-irc.org/.

Adversario, Patricia. 2003. Nurses' exodus making health systems sick. Inter Press Service. 15 May. http://ipsnews.net/.

Agathangelou, Anna. 2004. *The global political economy of sex: Desire, violence and insecurity in Mediterranean nation-states*. New York: Palgrave-Macmillan.

Agustin, Laura M. 2003. A migrant world of services. *Social Politics* 10, 3: 377-96.

—. 2007. *Sex at the margins: Migration, labour markets and the rescue industry*. London: Zed Books.

Alboim, Naomi, and Maytree. 2009. *Adjusting the balance: Fixing Canada's economic immigration policies*. http://www.maytree.com/.

Allen, Anita. 2003. *Why privacy isn't everything: Feminist reflections on personal accountability*. Lanham, MD: Roman and Littlefield.

Amoore, Louise. 2002. *Globalisation contested: An international political economy of work*. Manchester and New York: Manchester University Press.

Anderson, James, and Ian Shuttleworth. 2004. A new spatial fix for capitalist crisis? Immigrant labour, state borders and the new ostracizing imperialism. In *Global regulation: Managing crises after the imperial turn,* ed. Kees van der Pijl, Libby Assassi, and Duncan Wigan, 145-61. Basingstoke: Palgrave-Macmillan.

Antonnen, Anneli, and Jorma Sipilä. 1997. Europeanization of care services: Is it possible to identify models? *Journal of European Social Policy* 6, 2: 87-100.

Antonnen, Anneli, Jorma Sipilä, and John Baldock. 2003. *The young, the old and the state: Social care systems in five industrial nations.* Cheltenham: Edward Elgar.

Arat-Koc, Sedef. 2006. Whose social reproduction? Transnational motherhood and challenges to feminist political economy. In *Social reproduction: Feminist political economy challenges neoliberalism,* ed. Kate Bezanson and Meg Luxton, 75-92. Montreal and Kingston: McGill-Queen's University Press.

Armstrong, Pat, and Hugh Armstrong. 2008. *Health Care.* About Canada series. Halifax: Fernwood.

Asahi Shimbun. 2006. Nippi kyotei: Rodo kaikoku he aratana ippo [The Japan-Philippine agreement: A new step toward opening Japan's labour market]. 26 September.

–. 2008. Kaigo ni gaikokujin rodoryoku: Kadai ha [Foreign labour in care work: What are the issues?]. 11 February.

Asato Wako. 2007. Nippi keizai renkei kyotei to gaikokujin kaigoshi-kangoshi no ukeire [The reception of foreign nurses and care workers through the Japan-Philippine economic partnership agreement]. In *Kaigo-kaji rodosha no kokusai ido: Esunishitei-jienda-kea rodo no kosa* [The international transfers of care and domestic workers: The intersections of ethnicity, gender, and care labour], ed. Yoshiko Kuba, 27-50. Tokyo: Nihon Hyoron.

Asis, Maruja. 2006. Living with migration: Experiences of left-behind children in the Philippines. *Asian Population Studies* 2, 1: 45–67.

Bach, Stephen. 2003. International migration of health workers: Labour and social issues. Working Paper No. 209. Geneva: International Labour Office.

Bakan, Abigail, and Davia Stasiulis, eds. 1997. *Not one of the family: Foreign domestic workers in Canada.* Toronto: University of Toronto Press.

Bakker, Isabella. 1999. Neoliberal governance and the new gender order. *Working Papers* 1, 1: 49-59.

Bakker, Isabella, and Rachel Silvey. 2008. *Beyond states and markets: The challenges of social reproduction.* London: Routledge.

Baldassar, Loretta. 2007. Transnational families and aged care: The mobility of care and the migrancy of ageing. *Journal of Ethnic and Migration Studies* 33, 2: 275-97.

Baldock, C.V. 2000. Migrants and their parents: Care giving from a distance. *Journal of Family Issues* 21, 2: 205-24.

Ball, Rochelle E. 2004. Divergent development, racialized rights: Globalized labour markets and the trade of nurses – The case of the Philippines. *Women's Studies International Forum* 27, 2: 119-33.

–. 2008. Globalised labour markets and the trade of Filipino nurses: Implications for international regulatory governance. In *The internal migration of health workers,* ed. John Connell, 30-46. New York: Routledge.

Barber, Paul Gardiner. 2000. Agency in Philippine women's labour migration and provisional diaspora. *Women's Studies International Forum* 23, 4: 399-411.

Barker, Drucilla K. 2005. Beyond women and economics: Rereading "women's work." *Signs: Journal of Women in Culture and Society* 30, 4: 2189-209.

Batata, Amber S. 2005. International nurse recruitment and NHS vacancies: A cross-sectional analysis. *Globalization and Health* 1, 7: 1-7.

Baumann, Andrea, Jennifer Blythe, Camille Kolotylo, and Jane Underwood. 2004. *Immigration and emigration trends: A Canadian perspective*. Toronto: Nursing Sector Study Corporation.

Baumann, Andrea, Jennifer Blythe, Anne Rheaume, and Karen McIntosh. 2006. *Internationally educated nurses in Ontario: Maximizing the brain gain*. Human Health Resources Series Number 3. Ontario: Nursing Health Services Research Unit.

Bedford, Kate. 2008. Governing intimacy in the World Bank. In *Global governance: Feminist perspectives*, ed. Shirin Rai and Georgina Waylen, 1-18. London: Palgrave Macmillan.

–. 2009. Gender and institutional strengthening: The World Bank's policy record in Latin America. *Contemporary Politics* 15, 2: 197-214.

Bell, Daniel A. 2001. Equal rights for foreign resident workers? *Dissent* 48, 4: 26-34.

Benería, L., and M. Floro. 2006. Distribution, gender and labor market informalization: A conceptual framework with a focus on homeworkers. In *Gender and social policy in a global context: Uncovering the gendered structure of "the social,"* ed. S. Razawi and S. Hassim, 9-27. Basingstoke: Palgrave-Macmillan.

Beneria, Lourdes. 2003. *Gender, development and globalization: Economics as if people mattered*. New York: Routledge.

–. 2008. The crisis of care, international migration and public policy. *Feminist Economics* 14, 3: 1-21.

Benhabib, Seyla. 2004. *The rights of others*. Cambridge: Cambridge University Press.

Bennett, Colin J. 1991. How states utilize foreign evidence. *Journal of Public Policy* 11, 1: 31-54.

Bennett, John. 2008. *Benchmarks for early childhood services in OECD countries*. Florence: Innocenti Research Centre of UNICEF.

Bettio, F., A. Simonazzi, and P. Villa. 2006. Change in care regimes and female migration: The care drain in the Mediterranean. *Journal of European Social Policy* 16, 3: 271-85.

Bezanson, Kate, and Meg Luxton. 2006. Introduction: Social reproduction and feminist political economy. In *Social reproduction: Feminist political economy challenges neo-liberalism*, ed. Kate Bezanson and Meg Luxton, 3-10. Montreal and Kingston: McGill-Queen's University Press.

Bilefsky, Dan. 2009. Czechs cool to presence of workers from Asia. *New York Times*, 7 June.

Blyth, Mark. 2002. *Great transformations: Economic ideas and institutional change in the twentieth century*. Cambridge: Cambridge University Press.

Blythe, Jennifer, and Andrea Baumann. 2009. Internationally educated nurses: Profiling workforce diversity. *International Nursing Review* 56: 191-97.

Boling, Patricia. 1998. Family policy in Japan. *Journal of Social Policy* 27, 2: 173-90.

–. 2003. Political explanations for Japanese family policies. Paper prepared for the International Sociological Association annual meeting of the research committee on poverty, social welfare, and social policy, 21-24 August, Toronto.

Boone, J. 2007. Nord Anglia sells nurseries to ABC. *Financial Times*, 14 August.

Bosniak, Linda. 2009. Citizenship, noncitizenship, and the transnationlization of domestic work. In *Migrations and mobilities: Citizenship, borders, and gender*, ed. Seyla Benhabib and Judith Resnik, 127-56. New York: New York University Press.

Boyd, Monica, and Deanna Pikkov. 2008. Finding a place in stratified structures. In *New perspectives on gender and migration*, ed. Nicola Piper, 19-58. New York: UNRISD.

Bråten, Stein. 2003. Participant perception of others' acts: Virtual otherness in infants and adults. *Culture and Psychology* 9, 3: 261-76.

Brennan, D. 2007. The ABC of child care politics. *Australian Journal of Social Issues* 42, 2: 213-55.

Brown, S. 2006. Can remittances spur development? A critical survey. *International Studies Review* 8, 1: 55-75.

Brown, Wendy. 2005. *Edgework: Critical essays on knowledge and politics*. Princeton, NJ: Princeton University Press.

Bruckert, C., and C. Parent. 2002. *Trafficking in human beings and organized crime: A Literature Review*. RCMP research and evaluation branch, community, contract and aboriginal policing service directorate. http://www.rcmp-grc.gc.ca/.

Buchan, James, and Lynn Calman. 2004. *The global shortage of registered nurses: An overview of issues and actions*. Geneva: International Council of Nurses.

Cabinet Office (Japan). 2002a. *Kokumin seikatsu hakusho* [White paper on the national lifestyle]. Tokyo, Japan: Kokuritsu Insatsukyoku. http://www5.cao.go.jp/.

–. 2002b. Kokumin seikatsu ni kansuru seron chōsa [Opinion poll on the national lifestyle]. http://www8.cao.go.jp/.

–. 2003. Kōreisha kaigo ni kansuru seron chōsa [Opinion poll on elderly care]. http://www8.cao.go.jp/.

–. 2004. *Shōshika shakai hakusho* [White paper on the declining birthrate]. Tokyo: Gyōsei.

–. 2006a. Aratana shōshika taisaku ni tsuite [Memo on new measures for increasing the birthrate]. http://www.keizai-shimon.go.jp/.

–. 2006b. Dai 10-kai shōshika shakai taisak suishin senmon iinkai [Minutes of the 10th advisory panel on the promotion of measures for reversing the declining birthrate]. http://www8.cao.go.jp/.

–. 2008a. *Shōshika shakai hakusho* [White paper on the declining birthrate]. Tokyo: Gyōsei.

–. 2008b. *White paper on aging society 2007*. http://www8.cao.go.jp/. Tokyo: Cabinet Office.

Campbell, John L. 2002. Ideas, politics, and public policy. *Annual Review of Sociology* 28: 21-38.

–, ed. 2004. *Institutional change and globalization.* Princeton: Princeton University Press.

Canadian Institute for Health Information (CIHI). 2007. *Internationally educated physicians and nurses in Canada.* http://secure.cihi.ca/.

Cancedda, A., ed. 2001. *Employment in household services.* Dublin: European Foundation for the Improvement of Living and Working Conditions.

Card, Claudia. 2002. Responsibility ethics, shared understandings, and moral communities. *Hypatia* 17, 1: 141-55.

Carens, Joseph H. 2008a. Live-in domestics, seasonal workers, and others hard to locate on the map of democracy. *Journal of Political Philosophy* 16, 4: 419-45.

–. 2008b. The rights of irregular migrants. *Ethics and International Affairs* 22: 163-86.

Carnegie Task Force on Meeting the Needs of Young Children. 1994. *Starting points.* New York: Carnegie Corporation.

Carse, Alisa L., and Hilde Lindemann Nelson. 1996. Rehabilitating care. *Kennedy Institute of Ethics Journal* 6, 1: 19-35.

Castles, Stephen. 2005. Nation and empire: Hierarchies of citizenship in the new global order. *International Politics* 42, 2: 203-24.

CCR (Canadian Council for Refugees). 2008. Comments on the Canadian experience class proposal. http://ccrweb.ca/.

Chang, Grace. 2000. *Disposable domestics: Immigrant women workers in the global economy.* Cambridge: South End Press.

Chang, Grace, and Kathleen Kim. 2007. Reconceptualizing approaches to human trafficking: New directions and perspectives from the field(s). *Stanford Journal of Civil Rights and Civil Liberties* 3, 2: 318-44.

Chang, Kimberly A., and L.H.M. Ling. 2000. Globalization and its intimate other: Filipina domestic workers in Hong Kong. In *Gender and global restructuring: Sightings, sites and resistances*, ed. Marianne H. Marchand and Anne Sisson Runyan, 27-43. London and New York: Routledge.

Cherninska, T. 2007. Zhinocha migracia: Zmina gendernyh rolej [Female migration. Change of gender roles]. Fond suspil'noj bezpeky [Societal security fund]. http://fsb.net.ua/.

Cho, W.H. 2005. Productive welfare: Welfare of Korea. In *A new paradigm for social welfare in the new millennium*, ed. Lee-Jay Cho, Hyungpyo Moon, Yoon Hyung Kim, and Sang-Hyop Lee, 55-98. Seoul: Korea Development Institute.

Chodorow, Nancy. 1978. *The reproduction of mothering.* Berkeley: University of California Press.

Choi, Eunyoung. 2008. New social risks in Korea: Balancing work and family, income polarization. Paper presented at Trilateral Social Policy Research Project Health Care, Work-Family Responsibilities and Income Redistribution in Diversified and Aging Societies, 16-17 February, Tokyo, Japan.

Choi, Kyungsoo. 2009. Social cohesion (4): Korea's social cohesion – issues and prospects. *Korea Herald*, 12 August. Analysis section. http://www.koreaherald.co.kr/.

Chosun Daily. 2007. Family Ministry to offer low-cost nanny care. 5 April.

Citizenship and Immigration Canada (CIC). 2008a. *Annual report to Parliament on immigration 2008*. http://www.cic.gc.ca/.

–. 2008b. Canada's government to help temporary foreign workers and foreign student graduates become permanent residents. News release, 12 August. http://www.cic.gc.ca/.

–. 2009. *Eligibility criteria for federal skilled worker applications*. http://www.cic.gc.ca/.

Code, Lorraine. 2002. Narratives of responsibility and agency: Reading Margaret Walker's moral understandings. *Hypatia* 17, 1: 156-73.

Connell, John, ed. 2008. *The international migration of health workers*. New York: Routledge.

Connell, R.W., and James W. Messerschmidt. 2005. Hegemonic masculinity: Rethinking the concept. *Gender and Society* 19, 6: 829-59.

Cornelius, Wayne, Takeyuki Tsuda, Philip Martin, and James Hollifield, eds. 2004. *Controlling immigration: A global perspective*. 2nd ed. Stanford: Stanford University Press.

Craig, David, and Doug Porter. 2004. The third way and the third world: Poverty reduction and social inclusion in the rise of "inclusive" liberalism. *Review of International Political Economy* 11, 2: 226-63.

Crisp, N. 2007. *Global health partnerships: The UK contribution to health in developing countries*. London: Central Office for Information.

Dahlberg, Gunilla, and Peter Moss. 2008. Beyond quality in early childhood education and care: Languages of evaluation. *CESifo DICE Report* 6, 2: 21-28. http://www.cesifo-group.de/.

Daly, Mary, and Jane Lewis. 2000. The concept of social care and the analysis of contemporary welfare states. *British Journal of Sociology* 51, 2: 281-98.

Daly, Mary. 2002. Care as good for social policy. *Journal of Social Policy* 31, 2: 251-70.

Datta, Kavita, Cathy McIlwaine, Jane Wills, Yara Evans, Joanna Herbert, and Jon May. 2007. The new development finance or exploiting migrant labour: Remittance sending among low-paid workers in London. *International Development Planning Review* 29, 1: 43-67.

Davies, Matt, and Michael Niemann. 2002. The everyday spaces of global politics: Work, leisure, family. *New Political Economy* 24, 4: 557-77.

Deacon, Bob. 2007. *Global social policy and governance*. London: Sage.

Deacon, Bob, and Alexandra Kaasch. 2008. The OECD's social and health policy: Neoliberal stalking horse or balancer of social and economic objectives? In *The OECD and transnational governance*, ed. Rianne Mahon and Stephen McBride, 226-41. Vancouver: UBC Press.

Detlev, L. 2009. Research note: Job mobilities and family lives in Europe. *Cosmobilities Newsletter* 4, 1: 2.

Devas, Cora. 2007. *Human trafficking true stories: A view of the world and everyone in it*. http://crudelia.wordpress.com/.

DfID (Department for International Development). 2006. UK helping to slow down "brain drain" that costs African lives. http://www.dfid.gov.uk/.

DiQuinzio, Patrice, and Iris Marion Young. 1995. Introduction: Special issue on feminist ethics and social policy. *Hypatia* 10, 1: 1-7.

Dobrowolsky, A., and J. Jenson. 2004. Shifting representations of citizenship: Canadian politics of "women" and "children." *Social Politics* 11, 2: 154-80.

Dovzhenko, Valentine. 2001. Introduction. In *Social work in prevention of human trafficking and protection of victims*, 3-4. Kyiv: Ukrainian Institute of Social Studies Press.

Dudwick, Nora, Radhika Srinivasan, and Jeanine Braithwaite. 2002. Ukraine gender review. Washington, DC: ECSSD. http://siteresources.worldbank.org/.

Duffy, Mignon. 2005. Reproducing labor inequalities: Challenges for feminists conceptualizing care at the intersections of gender, race, and class. *Gender and Society* 19, 1: 66-82.

Dumont, Jean-Christophe, Pascal Zurn, Jody Church, and Christine Le Thi. 2008. International mobility of health professionals and health workforce management in Canada: Myths and realities. OECD Health Working Paper No. 40, Paris, OECD.

Dworkin, Ronald. 2000. *Sovereign virtue: The theory and practice of equality*. Cambridge, MA: Harvard University Press.

ECLAC (Economic Commission for Latin America and the Caribbean). 2007. *Social cohesion: Inclusion and a sense of belonging in Latin America and the Caribbean*. New York: United Nations.

Ehrenreich, Barbara. 2000. Maid to order: The politics of other women's work. *Harper's Magazine*, 30, 1799: 59-70.

Ehrenreich, Barbara, and Arlie R. Hochschild, eds. 2002. *Global women: Nannies, maids, and sex workers in the new economy*. New York: Holt.

Elson, D. 2004. Social policy and macroeconomic performance: Integrating "the economic" and "the social." In *Social policy in a development context*, ed. Thandika Mkandawire, 63-79. Geneva: UNRISD/Palgrave-Macmillan.

Engster, Daniel. 2005. Rethinking care theory: The practice of caring and the obligation to care. *Hypatia* 20, 3: 50-74.

Esping-Andersen, Gøsta. 1990. *Three worlds of welfare capitalism*. Princeton University: Princeton University Press.

–. 1999. *Social foundations of postindustrial economies*. Oxford: Oxford University Press.

Esping-Andersen, Gøsta, Duncan Gallie, Anton Hemerijk, and John Myers. 2002. *Why we need a new welfare state*. Oxford: Oxford University Press.

Eto, Mikiko. 2001a. Public involvement in social policy reform: Seen from the perspective of Japan's elderly-care insurance scheme. *Journal of Social Policy* 30, 1: 17-36.

–. 2001b. Women's leverage on social policymaking in Japan. *PS: Political Science and Politics* 34, 2: 241-46.

Eviota, Elizabeth Uy. 1992. *The political economy of gender: Women and the sexual division of labour in the Philippines*. London and New York: Zed.

EWL (European Women's Lobby). 1995. *Confronting the fortress: Black and migrant women in the European Union*. Brussels, European Parliament, Directorate General for Research.

–. 2007. *Equal rights equal voices: Migrant women in the European Union.* http://www.womenlobby.org/.
Folbre, Nancy. 1994. *Who pays for the kids? Gender and the structure of constraint.* New York: Routledge.
–. 2001. *The invisible heart: Economics and family values.* New York: New Press.
–. 2006. The invisible heart. In *Global dimensions of gender and care work*, ed. Mary K. Zimmerman, Jacquelyn S. Litt, and Christine E. Bose, 211-16. Stanford: Stanford University Press.
–. 2008. Reforming care. *Politics and Society* 36, 3: 373-87.
Folbre, Nancy, and Julie A. Nelson. 2000. For love or money – or both. *Journal of Economic Perspectives* 14, 4: 123-40.
Fraser, Nancy. 1989a. Talking about needs: Interpretive contests as political conflict in welfare-state societies. *Ethics* 99, 2: 291-313.
–. 1989b. *Unruly practices: Power, discourse, and gender in contemporary social theory.* Minneapolis: University of Minnesota Press.
–. 1997. *Justice interruptus: Critical reflections on the "postsocialist" condition.* New York: Routledge.
–. 2008. Social rights and gender justice in the neoliberal moment: A conversation about welfare and transnational politics. *Feminist Theory* 8, 9: 225-45.
Friedman, Elisabeth Joy. 2003. Gendering the agenda: The impact of the transnational women's rights movement at the UN conferences of the 1990s. *Women's Studies International Forum* 26, 4: 313-31.
Gabriel, Christina. 2004. A question of skills: Gender, migration policy and the global political economy. In *Global Regulation: Managing crises after the imperial turn,* ed. Kees van der Pijl, Libby Assassi, and Duncan Wigan, 162-76. Basingstoke, UK: Palgrave.
–. 2008. A "healthy" trade? NAFTA, labour mobility and Canadian nurses. In *Governing international labour Migration,* ed. Christina Gabriel and Hélène Pellerin, 112-27. London: Routledge.
Galabuzi, Grace-Edward. 2005. Factors affecting the social economic status of Canadian immigrants in the new millennium. *Canadian Issues: Immigration and the Intersections of Diversity* (Spring): 53-60.
Galarneau, Diane. 2003. Health care professionals. In *Perspectives on labour and income.* Statistics Canada, cat. no. 75-001 4:5.
Garrett, Laurie. 2007. The challenge of global health. *Foreign Affairs* 86, 1: 14-38.
Gilligan, Carol. 1982. *In a different voice.* Cambridge, MA: Harvard University Press.
Glover, S., C. Gott, A. Loizillon, J. Porter, R. Price, S. Spencer, V. Srinivasan, and C. Willis. 2001. Migration: An economic and social analysis. RDS Occasional Paper No. 67. London: Home Office.
Goodhart, Michael. 2005. *Democracy as human rights: Freedom and equality in the age of globalization.* New York: Routledge.
Grasswick, Heide E. 2003. The impurities of epistemic responsibility: Developing a practice-oriented espistemology. In *Recognition, responsibility and rights: Feminist ethics and social theory,* ed. R.N. Fiore and H.L. Nelson, 89-104. Lanham, MD: Rowman and Littlefield.

Grinspun, D. 2003. Part-time and casual nursing work: The perils of healthcare restructuring. *International Journal of Sociology and Social Policy* 23, 8-9: 54-80.
Groenhout, Ruth E. 2004. *Connected lives: Human nature and an ethics of care*. Lanham, MD: Rowman and Littlefield.
Haas, E. 1992. Introduction: Epistemic communities and international policy coordination. *International Organization* 46, 1: 1-35.
Hanami Tadashi, and Kuwabara Yasuo. 1989. *Asu no rinjin: Gaikokujin rodosha* [Tomorrow's neighbours: Foreign workers]. Tokyo: Toyo Keizai Shimpo.
Hankivsky, Olena. 2004. *Social policy and the ethic of care*. Vancouver: UBC Press.
–. 2006. Imagining ethical globalization: The contributions of a care ethic. *Journal of Global Ethics* 2, 1: 91-110.
–. 2008. Gender, globalization and sex trafficking in Ukraine. In *Global science/Women's health*, ed. Cindy Patton and Helen Loshny. Youngstown, NY: Cambrian Press.
Hankivsky, Olena, and Anastasiya Salnykova. Forthcoming. Gender mainstreaming in Ukraine. In *Gender, politics and society in Ukraine*, ed. O. Hankivsky and A. Salnykova. Toronto: University of Toronto Press.
Haskell, Thomas L. 1998. *Objectivity is not neutrality: Explanatory schemes in history*. Baltimore: Johns Hopkins University Press.
Hassim. S. 2006. Whose utopia? A response to Gornick and Meyers "Institutions that support egalitarianism in parenthood and employment." Paper presented at the Real Utopias Conference, University of Wisconsin, Madison. http://www.ssc.wisc.edu/.
Health Canada. 2009. Commission on the Future of Health Care in Canada (Romanov Commission). http://www.hc-sc.gc.ca/.
Heckman, J.J. 1999. Policies to foster human capital. Paper presented at the Aaron Wildavsky Forum, University of California, Berkeley.
Held, Virginia. 1993. *Feminist morality: Transforming culture, society and politics*. Chicago: University of Chicago Press.
–. 2002. Care and the extension of markets. *Hypatia* 17, 2: 19-33.
–. 2006. *The ethics of care: Personal, political, and global*. Oxford: Oxford University Press.
Henninger, Annette, Christine Wimbauer, and Rosine Dombrowski. 2008. Demography as a push toward gender equality? Current reforms of German family policy. *Social Politics* 15, 3: 287-314.
Heymann, J., A. Earle, and A. Hanchate. 2004. Bringing a global perspective to community, work and family: An examination of extended work hours in families in four countries. *Community, Work and Family* 7, 2: 4.
High-Level Dialogue on International Migration and Development of the General Assembly of the United Nations. 2006. *Chairperson's summary of the high-level dialogue on international migration and development*. New York: United Nations.
Higuchi Keiko. 1999. Doukyo kazoku ni taisuru hōmon kaigo ni Kansuru Ikensho [The statement on the payment to family care-givers]. Paper presented at the 18th Joint Meeting of the Council of Medical Insurance and Welfare, 20 September, Toyko, Japan. http://www1.mhlw.go.jp/.

Himmelweit, Susan. 2008. Policy on care: A help or a hindrance to gender equality? In *Women and employment: Changing lives and new challenges*, ed. J. Scott, S. Dex, and H. Joshi, 347-68. Cheltenham, UK: Edward Elgar.

Hochschild, Adam. 2005. Bury the chains: Prophets and rebels in the fight to free an empire's slaves. New York: Houghton Mifflin.

Hochschild, Arlie Russell. 2000. Global care chains and emotional surplus value. In *Global capitalism*, ed. Will Hutton and Anthony Giddens, 130-46. New York: The New Press.

–. 2005. Love and gold. In *Feminist politics, activism, and vision: Local and global challenges*, ed. L. Ricciutelli, A.R. Miles, and M. McFadden, 34-46. London: Zed.

Holden, C. 2002. The internationalization of long-term care provision: Economics and strategy. *Global Social Policy* 2, 1: 47-67.

Honda Yuki. 2008. *Katei kyōiku no airo* [The gridlock of home education]. Tokyo: Keisō Shobō.

Hondagneu-Sotelo, Pierrette. 2000. The international division of caring and cleaning work. In *Care work, gender, labour and the welfare state*, ed. Madonna Harrington Meyer, 149-62. New York: Routledge.

–. 2001. *Doméstica: Immigrant workers cleaning and caring in the shadows of affluence.* Berkeley: University of California Press.

Hooper, Charlotte. 2000. Masculinities in transition: The case of globalization. In *Gender and global restructuring: Sightings, sites and resistances*, ed. Marianne H. Marchand and Anne Sisson Runyan, 59-73. London: Routledge.

Hoskyns, C. 1996. *Integrating gender: Women, law and politics in the European Union.* London: Verso.

Hughes, D.M., and T.A. Denisova. 2001. The transnational political criminal nexus of trafficking in women from Ukraine. *Trends in Organized Crime* 6, 3-4: 1-22.

Hulme, Rob. 2006. The role of policy transfer in assessing the impact of American ideas on British social policy. *Global Social Policy* 6, 2: 173-95.

Hutchings, Kimberley. 2000. Towards a feminist international ethics. *Review of International Studies* 26, 5: 111-30.

–. 2001. Ethics, feminism, and international affairs. In *Ethics and international affairs: Extent and limits*, ed. Jean-Marc Coicaud and Daniel Warner, 194-216. Tokyo: UN University Press.

Inoue Senichi. 2005. Kaigo bijinesu to gaikokujin rodosha [Nursing-care business and foreign workers]. *The Annals of Osaka University of Human Science* 4: 95-104.

International Centre for Human Resources in Nursing. 2008. *Workplace bullying in the health sector.* Geneva: International Centre for Human Resources in Nursing.

Ito Ruri, Ogaya Chiho, Tenegra Brenda, and Inaba Nanako. 2005. Ika ni shite "kea jozu na Fuiripinjin" ha tsukurareruka? Kea giba to sai seisan rodo no "kokusai shohin" ka [How are "caring Filipinos" made? Caregivers and the "international commodification" of reproductive labour]. *Frontiers of Gender Studies Journal* 3: 269-87.

Iversen, Torben, and Anne Wren. 1998. Equality, employment and budgetary restraint: The trilemma of the service economy. *World Politics* 50, 4: 507-46.

Jackson, Andrew. 2008. Crafting the conventional economic wisdom: The OECD and the Canadian policy process. In *The OECD and transnational governance*, ed. Rianne Mahon and Stephen McBride, 170-87. Vancouver: UBC Press.

Jeans, Mary Ellen, Fran Hadley, Jill Green, and Christine Da Prat. 2005. *Navigating to become a nurse in Canada: Assessment of international nurse applicants.* Ottawa: Canadian Nurses Association.

Jenson, Jane. 1986. Gender and reproduction: Or, babies and the state. *Studies in Political Economy* 20: 9-46.

–. 1997. Who cares? Gender and welfare regimes. *Social Politics* 4, 2: 182-87.

–. 2007. Redesigning citizenship regimes after neoliberalism: Ideas about social investment. Prepared for Research Committee 19, Florence, Italy. http://www.cccg.umontreal.ca/.

–. 2008. Diffusing ideas after neo-liberalism: The social investment perspective in Europe and Latin America. Paper presented at the 2008 meetings of Research Committee 19 of the International Sociology Association, Stockholm, Sweden.

Jenson, J., and D. Saint-Martin. 2006. Building blocks for a new social architecture: The LEGO TM paradigm of an active society. *Policy and Politics* 34, 3: 429-51.

Jolly, Richard. 1991. Adjustment with a human face: A UNICEF record and perspective on the 1980s. *World Development* 19, 12: 1807-21.

Jones, Phillip, and David Coleman. 2005. *The United Nations and education: Multilateralism, development and globalisation.* London and New York: Routledge.

Jones, Rochelle. 2005. Trafficking of women in Eastern Europe: An interview with La Strada-Ukraine on their program for the prevention of trafficking of women from Central and Eastern Europe. http://www.socialniprava.info/.

Joo, Sungsoo, Seonmi Lee, and Youngjae Jo. 2006. *The explosion of CSOs and citizen participation: An assessment of civil society in South Korea 2004.* CIVICUS Civil Society Index Report for South Korea.

Kabeer, Naila. 1994. *Reversed realities: Gender hierarchies in development.* London, UK: Verso.

Kalayaan and Oxfam. 2008. *The new bonded labor: The impact of proposed changes to the UK immigration system on migrant domestic workers.* London: Oxfam and Kalayaan.

Kamerman, Sheila B. 2006. A global history of early childhood education and care. Background paper prepared for *Education for all global monitoring report 2007: Strong foundations – Early childhood care and education.* Paris: UNESCO.

Kardam, Nüket. 2004. The emerging global gender equality regime from neoliberal and constructivist perspectives in international relations. *International Feminist Journal of Politics* 6, 1: 88-109.

Katz, C. 2001. Vagabond capitalism and the necessity for social reproduction. *Antipode* 33: 707-28.

Kawano Yukio. 2007. Zainichi Korian no koreika to esunishitei [The aging of Korean-Japanese and ethnicity]. In *Ibunka kan kaigo to tabunka kyosei: Dare ga kaigo o ninaunoka* [Elder care in a multicultural society: Who shoulders elder care?], ed. Chizuko Kawamura and Won-sok Son, 118-47. Tokyo: Akashi.

Keefe, Janice, and Beth Rajnovich. 2007. To pay or not to pay: Examining underlying principles in the debate on financial support for family caregivers. *Canadian Journal on Aging* 26, 1: 77-90.

Kempadoo, Kamala. 2005. From moral panic to global justice: Changing perspectives on trafficking. In *Trafficking and prostitution reconsidered: New perspectives on migration, sex work and human rights*, ed. Kamala Kempadoo, vii-xxxiv. Boulder: Paradigm.

Kempadoo, Kamala, Jyoti Sanghera, and Bandana Pattanaik, eds. 2005. Introduction to *Trafficking and prostitution reconsidered: New perspectives on migration, sex work, and human rights*. Boulder: Paradigm Publishers.

Kershaw, Paul, Jane Pulkingham, and Sylvia Fuller. 2008. Expanding the subject: Violence, care and (in)active male citizenship. *Social Politics* 15, 2: 182-206.

Keung, N. 2008. "New migrant class draws few." *Toronto Star*, 24 November.

Kibe, Takashi. 2006. Differential citizenship and ethnocultural groups: A Japanese case. *Citizenship Studies* 10, 4: 413-30.

Kikuchi Izumi. 2010. *Kazoku kaigo heno genkin shiharai* [Cash payments for family care]. Tokyo: Koshokuken.

Kim, Won-jong. 2007. Social investment and health and welfare policies. Paper presented at the Special Seminar of the Korean Association for Local Finance, April, Seoul, Korea.

Kim, Yeon-myung. 2007. Social investment strategy in Korea: Possibilities, issues and prospects. Paper presented at Conference on Social Investment Strategy, Seoul Welfare Foundation, 16 November, Seoul, Korea.

Kingma, Mireille. 2006. *Nurses on the move: Migration and the global health care economy*. Ithaca, NY: Cornell University Press.

Kittay, Eva. 2005. Dependency, difference and a global ethic of long-term care. *Journal of Political Philosophy* 13, 2: 443-69.

Klein, Naomi. 2007. *The shock doctrine: The rise of disaster capitalism*. New York: Henry Holt.

Kloer, A. 2009. No good jobs: Sokha and Makara's true story of slavery. *Change.org*. http://humantrafficking.change.org/.

Kofman, Eleonore. 2004. Gendered global migrations. *International Feminist Journal of Politics* 6, 4: 643-65.

—. 2008. Managing migration and citizenship in Europe: Towards an overarching framework. In *Governing International Labour Migration*, ed. Christina Gabriel and Hélène Pellerin, 13-26. London: Routledge.

Kofman, E., P. Raghuram, and M. Merefield. 2005. Gendered migrations: Towards gender sensitive policies in the UK. Asylum and Migration Working Paper No 6. London: Institute for Public Policy Research.

Kofman, E., and P. Raghuram. 2006. Gender and global labour migrations: Incorporating skilled workers. *Antipode* 38, 2: 282-303.

—. 2007. The implications of migration for gender and care regimes in the south. Paper prepared for UNRISD-IOM-IFS workshop on social policy and migration in developing countries, 22-23 November, Stockholm, Sweden. http://www.unrisd.org/.

—. 2009. The Implications of migration for gender and care regimes in the south. Social Policy and Development Programme Paper No. 41. Switzerland, UNRISD.
Koggel, Christine M. 1998. *Perspectives on equality: Constructing a relational theory.* Latham, MD: Rowman and Littlefield.
—. 2006a. Global inequalities and relational ethics. Paper presented at the annual meeting of the American Political Science Association. Philadelphia, PA.
—. ed. 2006b. *Moral issues in global perspective: Human diversity and equality.* 2nd ed. Vol. 2. Toronto: Broadview.
Kolawole, B. 2009. Ontario's internationally educated nurses and waste in human capital. *International Nursing Review* 56, 2: 184-90.
Korea Foundation for Working Together. 2008. *Annual report.* http://eng.hamkke.org/.
Korea Net. 2006. Childcare leave to extend to 3 years. http://www.korea.net/.
Kuba, Yoshiko. 2007. Preface. In *Kaigo-kaji rodosha no kokusai ido: Esunishitei-jienda-kea rodo no kosa* [The international transfers of care and domestic workers: The intersections of ethnicity, gender, and care labour], ed. Yoshiko Kuba, i-v. Tokyo: Nihon Hyoron.
Kurian, Rachel. 2006. The globalisation of domestic care services. In *Engendering human security: Feminist perspectives,* ed. Thanh-Dam Truong, Saskia Wieringa, and Amrita Chhachhi, 147-67. London: Zed Press.
KWDI (Korean Women's Development Institute). 2008. *Statistical handbook 2008: Women in Korea.* Seoul: KWDI
Kyzyma, I. 2007. *Female migration in Ukraine: Determinants and consequences.* Kirovohrad: Department of Economic Theory and Law.
Lakiza-Sachuk, N. 2003. Trafficking in women from Ukraine as a security issue. Paper presented at the Hawaii International Conference on Social Sciences, 12-15 December, Honolulu, Hawaii. (Publication of the Transnational Crime and Corruption Centre.)
Langevin, Louise, and Marie-Claude Belleau. 2000. *Trafficking in women in Canada: A critical analysis of the legal framework governing immigrant live-in caregivers and mail-order brides.* Ottawa: Status of Women Canada.
Lawson, Victoria. 2007. Geographies of care and responsibility. *Annals of the Association of American Geographers* 97, 1: 1-11.
Lee, Hyekyung. 2007. Future direction of social services in Korea. Keynote speech delivered at international symposium entitled Social Service Provision System: The Issues of Public-Private Partnership in Korea, 11-12 December, Seoul, Korea.
Lee Kunsun. 2007. Zainichi Korian koreisha no kaigo no genjo to kadai [The current conditions and issues of care for the aged Korean-Japanese]. In *Ibunka kan kaigo to tabunka kyosei: Dare ga kaigo o ninaunoka* [Elder care in a multicultural society: Who shoulders elder care?], ed. Chizuko Kawamura and Won-sok Son, 150-82. Tokyo: Akashi.
Lefebvre, Henri. 1991 [1974]. *The production of space.* Trans. Donald Nicholson-Smith. Oxford: Blackwell.
—. 1991 [1947]. *Critique of everyday life.* Trans. John Moore. London and New York: Verso.

Leitner, Sigrid. 2003. Varieties of familialism: The caring function of the family in comparative perspective. *European Societies* 5, 4: 353-75.

Levchenko, Kateryna. 1999. Combat of trafficking in women for the purpose of forced prostitution: Ukraine, country report. Vienna: Ludwig Boltzmann Institute of Human Rights. http://www.uri.edu/.

Levchenko, K., and O. Bandurko. 2006. Trudova mihratsiya ta protydiya torhivli liudmy [Labour migration and trafficking prevention]. Kiev: Yurystkonsult.

Levchenko, K., and I. Schvab. 2008. *Labor migration from Ukraine, Belarus, and Moldova to Russian Federation: Trends and connection with human trafficking.* Kiev: Agency Ukraine Ltd.

Levchenko, K., I. Schvab, E. Malinovskaya, and O. Trofimenko. 2010. Ukrainskaya Gretsiya: Prichiny, problem, perspektivy [Ukrainian Greece: Causes, problems, prospects]. Kiev: Instytut Sotsiologiyi NANU.

Levy, Traci M. 2005. At the intersection of intimacy and care: Redefining "family" through the lens of a public ethic of care. *Politics and Gender* 1, 1: 65-95.

Lewis, Jane. 2008. Work-family balance policies: Issues and developments in the United Kingdom, 1997-2005, in comparative perspective. In *Women and employment: Changing lives and new challenges*, ed. Jacqueline Scott, Shirley Dex, and Heather Joshi, 268-88. Cheltenham, UK: Edward Elgar Publishing.

Lewis, Jane, and Iona Ostner. 1991. Gender and the evolution of European social policies. Paper presented at the CES workshop entitled Emergent Supranational Social Policy: The EC's Social Dimension in Comparative Perspective, Harvard University, Centre for European Studies, Cambridge, MA.

Lister, Ruth. 1994. Dilemmas in engendering citizenship. *Economy and Society* 24, 1: 35-40.

Lister, Ruth, Fiona Williams, Anneli Antonnen, Jet Bussemaker, Ute Gerhard, Jacqueline Heinen, Stina Johansson, Arnlaug Leira, Birte Siim, Constanza Tobio, and Anna Gavanas. 2007. *Gendering citizenship in Western Europe: New challenges for citizenship research in a cross-national context.* Bristol: Policy Press.

Litt, Jacqueline, and Mary Zimmerman. 2003. Global perspectives on gender and carework: An introduction. *Gender and Society* 17, 2: 156-65.

Little, Lisa. 2007. Nurse migration: A Canadian case study. *Health Services Research* 42, 3: 1336-53.

Long, Susan Orpett, and Phyllis Braudy Harris. 2000. Gender and elder care: Social change and the role of the caregiver in Japan. *Social Science Japan Journal* 3, 1: 21-36.

Lorde, Audre. 1984. *Sister outsider: Essays and speeches.* Rumansburg, NY: Crossing Press.

Lutz, Helma. 2008. *Migration and domestic work: A European perspective on a global theme.* Surrey, UK: Ashgate.

Macedo, Stephen, Y. Alex-Assensoh, J.M. Berry, M. Brintnall, D.E. Campbell, L.R. Fraga, A. Fung, W.A. Galston, C.F. Karpowitz, M. Levi, M. Levinson, K. Lipsitz, R.G. Niemi, R.D. Putnam, W.M. Rahn, R. Reich, R.R. Rodgers, T. Swanstrom, and K.C. Walsh. 2005. *Democracy at risk: How political choices undermine citizen participation and what we can do about it.* Washington: Brookings Institution.

Macklin, Audrey. 2002. Public entrance/private member. In *Privatization, law, and the challenge to feminism*, ed. Brenda Cossman and Judy Fudge, 218-64. Toronto: University of Toronto Press.
—. 2003. Dancing across borders: Exotic dancers trafficking and Canadian immigration policy. *International Migration Review* 37, 2: 464-500.
Maher, Kristen Hill. 2004. Globalized social reproduction: Women migrants and the citizenship gap. In *People out of place: Globalization, human rights, and the citizenship gap*, ed. Alison Brysk and Gershon Shafir, 131-52. New York: Routledge.
Mahon, Rianne. 2006a. The OECD and the work/family reconciliation agenda: Competing frames. In *Children, changing families and welfare states*, ed. Jane Lewis, 173-97. Cheltenham, UK: Edward Elgar.
—. 2006b. Varieties of liberalism: Canadian social policy from the "golden age" to the "present." Paper presented at Multi-Pillar Systems of Social Safety Nets, an international conference sponsored by the Korea Development Institute and the World Bank, 24 November, Seoul, Korea.
—. 2009. The OECD's discourse on the reconciliation of work and family life. *Global Social Policy* 9, 2: 183-201.
—. 2010a. Early childhood education and care policies around the world: The impact of international organisations. In *The Routledge international handbook of early childhood education*, ed. Tony Bertram, John Bennett, Philip Gammage, and Christine Pascal. London: Routledge.
—. 2010b. Learning, forgetting, rediscovering: The OECD's "new" family policy. In *Mechanisms of OECD governance: International incentives for national policy making?*, ed. K. Martens and Anja Jakobi, 198-216. New York: Oxford University Press.
Mahon, Rianne, and Stephen McBride, eds. 2008. *The OECD and transnational governance*. Vancouver: UBC Press.
Mainichi Shimbun. 2008a. Indoneshiajin ukeire: Kaigo genba to seifu zure [The introduction of Indonesians: The gap between care-giving sites and the state's view]. 20 April. http://mainichi.jp/.
—. 2008b. Kea kaikoku: Indoneshia kaigoshi shinpai ha kenshugo no seikatsu [The opening of the country for care: Indonesian care workers, their concern is the life after training]. 19 November. http://mainichi.jp/.
Malarek, Victor. 2003. *The Natashas: Inside the new global sex trade*. Toronto: Penguin Books.
Malynovska, Olena. 2009. Caught between east and west, Ukraine struggles with its migration policy. Migration Policy Institute. http://www.migrationinformation.org/.
Marshall, T.H. 1998 [1963]. Citizenship and social class. Reprinted in *The citizenship debates*, ed. Gershon Shafir, 93-111. Minneapolis: University of Minnesota Press.
Mayo, M. 2005. *Global citizens: Social movements and the challenge of globalization*. London: Zed Press.
McBride, Stephen. 2001. *Paradigm shift: Globalization and the Canadian state*. Halifax: Fernwood.

McIntosh, Mary. 1978. The state and the oppression of women. In *Feminism and materialism,* ed. A. Kuhn and A. Wolpe, 254-89. London: Routledge.

McLaughlin, E., and C. Glendinning. 1994. Paying for care in Europe: Is there a feminist approach? In *Family policies and the welfare of women,* ed. L. Hantrais and S. Mangen. Loughborough: Cross-National Research Group.

McNeil-Walsh, Colleen. 2008. Migrant nurses and the experience of skill: South African nurses in the UK health care sector. In *The international migration of health workers,* ed. John Connell, 129-46. New York: Routledge.

METI (Ministry of Economy, Trade and Industry, Japan). 2006. Global Economic Strategy. April. http://www.meti.go.jp/.

Meyer, John W., John Boli, George M. Thomas, and Francisco O. Ramirez. 1997. World society and the nation-state. *American Journal of Sociology* 103, 1: 144-81.

Meyer, Madonna Harrington, ed. 2000. *Care work: Gender, labor and the welfare state.* New York: Routledge.

MHLW (Ministry of Health, Labour, and Welfare, Japan). 2003a. Dai 23-kai rōdō seisaku shingikai koyō kintō bunkakai [Minutes of the 23rd meeting of the Committee of Equal Employment in the Labour Policy Council]. http://www.mhlw.go.jp/.

–. 2003b. Dai 28-kai rōdō seisaku shingikai koyō kintō bunkakai [Minutes of the 28th meeting of the Committee of Equal Employment in the Labour Council]. http://www.mhlw.go.jp/.

–. 2004. Kaigo yobō ni tsuite [On care prevention]. http://www.wam.go.jp/.

–. 2005a. Gaikokujin kaigo fukushishi no shugyo seigen no kanwa to [The liberation in the employment of foreign care workers, etc.]. March. http://www.mhlw.go.jp/.

–. 2005b. Kaigo kyūfuhi jittai chōsa geppō [Monthly report on LTCI provisioning]. http://www-bm.mhlw.go.jp/.

–. 2006. Keizai jo no teikei ni kansuru Nihon koku to Fuiripin kyowakoku tono aida no kyotei ni motoduku kango oyobi kaigo bunya ni okeru Fuiripinjin kangoshi to no ukeire no jisshi ni kansuru shishin (an) [The (proposed) guide for the reception of Filipino nurses and care workers through the Economic Partnership Agreement between Japan and the Republic of the Philippines]. http://www.mhlw.go.jp/.

–. 2007a. Heisei 19 nen jinko dotai tokei no nenkan suikei [2007 annual vital statistics report]. http://www.mhlw.go.jp/.

–. 2007b. Shakai fukushishi oyobi kaigo fukushishi ho to no ichibu o kaisei suru horitsuan ni tsuite [About the bill for partial amendments to social welfare and care welfare laws]. http://www.mhlw.go.jp/.

MHW (Ministry of Health and Welfare, Japan). 1991. *Kōsei hakusyo* [Annual reports on health and welfare]. Tokyo: Kōsei Mondai Kenkyūkai.

Mill, John Stuart. 1998. *On liberty and other essays.* New ed. New York: Oxford.

Miller, David. 2008a. Immigrants, nations, and citizenship. *Journal of Political Philosophy* 16, 4: 371-90.

–. 2008b. Irregular migrants: An alternative perspective. *Ethics and International Affairs* 22, 2: 193-97.

Mills, Charles. 1997. *The racial contract*. Ithaca, NY: Cornell University Press.
Ministry of Labor (Korea). 2008. http://english.molab.go.kr/.
—. 1998. *Kōsei hakusyo* [Annual report on health and welfare]. Tokyo: Kōsei Mondai Kenkyūkai.
Ministry of Planning and Budget (Korea). 2007. *Vision 2030*. Seoul: Ministry of Planning and Budget.
Misra, Joya, Sabine Merz, and Jonathan Woodring. 2006. The globalization of care work: Neoliberal economic restructuring and migration policy. *Globalizations* 3, 3: 317-22.
MOFA (Ministry of Foreign Affairs, Japan). 2006. Agreement between Japan and the Republic of the Philippines for an economic partnership. September. http://www.mofa.go.jp/.
—. 2007a. Agreement between Japan and the Kingdom of Thailand for an economic partnership. April. http://www.mofa.go.jp/.
—. 2007b. Agreement between Japan and the Republic of Indonesia for an economic partnership. August. http://www.mofa.go.jp/.
—. 2011. Japan-Thailand economic partnership agreement: Annex 7 referred to in Chapter 9, Specific commitments for the movement of natural persons. January. http://www.mofa.go.jp/.
Molyneux, M. 2006. Mothers at the service of the new poverty agenda: Progresa/oportunidades, Mexico's conditional transfer programme. *Social Policy and Administration* 40, 4: 425-49.
Molyneux, M., and Razavi, S., eds. 2002. *Gender justice, development and rights*. Oxford: Oxford University Press/UNRISD.
Mori, Hiromi. 1997. *Immigration policy and foreign workers in Japan*. New York: St. Martin's Press.
Mullin, Amy. 2005. Trust, social norms, and motherhood. *Journal of Social Philosophy* 36, 3: 316-30.
Myers, Robert G. 1987. *The eleven who survive: Toward a re-examination of early childhood development program options and costs*. Washington, DC: The World Bank.
—. 1991. Child development programs in UNICEF: The next ten years. Prepared for UNICEF.
—. 2000. Early childhood care and development: A global review. Paris: UNESCO.
Na, Jung, and Mugyeong Moon. 2003. *Integrating policies and systems for early childhood education and care: The case of the Republic of Korea*. Paris: UNESCO (Early Childhood and Family Policy Series No. 7).
NIKKEIREN (Japan Federation of Employers' Association) and RENGO (Japanese Trade Union Confederation). 2000. Kodomo wo umi sodateyasui shakai wo mezashite [Aiming at a friendly society for childbirth and child rearing: The joint declaration on the issue of the declining birthrate]. http://www.nikkeiren.or.jp/.
Noddings, Nel. 1984. *Caring: A feminine approach to ethics and moral education*. Berkeley: University of California Press.
NSOK (National Statistics Office of Korea). 2002. *Report on social statistics Survey*. Seoul: NSO.

Nussbaum, Martha C. 1987. *Nature, function, and capability: Aristotle on political distribution.* Helsinki: World Institute for Development Economics Research of the United Nations University.
–. 2004. Beyond the social contract: Capabilities and global justice. *Oxford Development Studies* 32, 1: 3-18.
–. 2007. The Supreme Court, 2006 term, Foreword – Constitutions and capabilities: "Perception" against lofty formalism. *Harvard Law Review* 121, 4: 84-86.
O'Connell Davidson, Julia. 2006. Will the real sex slave please stand up? *Feminist Review* 83: 4-22.
O'Connor, Julia. 1993. Gender, class and citizenship in the comparative analysis of welfare state regimes: Theoretical and methodological issues. *British Journal of Sociology* 44, 3: 503-18.
OECD (Oganization for Economic Cooperation and Development). 1974. Care of children of working parents. Directorate for social affairs, manpower and education, social affairs and industrial relations division for the working party on the role of women in the economy. Paris: OECD.
–. 1994. New orientations for social policy. Social Policy Studies 12. Paris: OECD.
–. 2004. Early child education and care 2004: Country profiles – Korea. http://www.oecd.org/.
–. 2006. *Starting strong: Early childhood education and care.* Paris: OECD.
–. 2007. *Babies and bosses: Reconciling work and family life – A synthesis of findings for OECD countries.* Paris: OECD.
–. 2008. Growing unequal: Income distribution and poverty in OECD countries. Paris: OECD.
–. 2009. OECD family database. http://www.oecd.org/.
Orloff, Ann. 1993. Gender and the social rights of citizenship: The comparative analysis of gender relations and welfare states. *American Sociological Review* 58: 303-28.
Orozco, M., L. Lowell, and J. Schneider. 2006. *Gender-specific determinants of remittances: Differences in structures and motivation.* Report presented to the World Bank Group Gender and Development Group, Washington. http://siteresources.worldbank.org/.
Österle A., and E. Hammer. 2007. Care allowances and the formalization of care arrangements: The Austrian experience. In *Cash for care in developed welfare states,* ed. Clare Ungerson and Sue Yeandle, 32-59. Basingstoke: Palgrave.
Parreñas, Rhacel Salazar. 2000. Migrant Filipina domestic workers and the international division of reproductive labor. *Gender and Society* 14: 560-81.
–. 2001a. *Servants of globalization: Women, migration and domestic work.* Stanford: Stanford University Press.
–. 2001b. Transgressing the nation-state: The partial citizenship and "imagined (global) community" of migrant Filipina domestic workers. *Signs: Journal of Women in Culture and Society* 26, 4: 1129-54.
–. 2003. The care crisis in the Philippines: Children and transnational families in the new global economy. In *Global woman: Nannies, maids and sex workers in the new economy,* ed. Barbara Ehrenreich and Arlie Russell Hochschild, 39-54. New York: Henry Holt.

–. 2005a. *Children of global migration: Transnational families and gendered woes.* Stanford: Stanford University Press.
–. 2005b. The international division of reproductive labor: Paid domestic work and globalization. In *Critical globalization studies*, ed. Richard P. Appelbaum and William I. Robinson, 237-47. London and New York: Routledge.
Pateman, Carole, and Charles W. Mills. 2007. *Contract and domination.* Boston: Polity.
Payrow Shabani, Omid A. 2007. Cosmopolitan justice and immigration. *European Journal of Social Theory* 10: 87-98.
Pearson, R. 2004. The social is political: Toward the re-politicization of feminist analysis of the global economy. *International Feminist Journal of Politics* 6, 4: 603-22.
Peck, Jamie, and Nik Theodore. 2008. Recombinant workfare across the Americas. Paper presented at the annual meetings of the Association of American Geographers, March, Boston, MA.
Peng, Ito. 2002. Social care in crisis: Gender, demography, and welfare state restructuring in Japan. *Social Politics* 9, 3: 411-43.
–. 2004. Postindustrial pressures, political regime shifts, and social policy reform in Japan and South Korea. *Journal of East Asian Studies* 4: 389-425.
–. 2008. Welfare policy reforms in Japan and Korea: Cultural and institutional factors. In *Culture and welfare state: Values of social policy from a comparative perspective,* ed. Wim van Oorschot, Michael Opielka, and Birgit Pfau-Effinger, 162-84. London: Edward Elgar.
Peng, Ito, and Joseph Wong. 2008. Institutions and institutional purpose: Continuity and change in East Asian Social Policy. *Politics and Society* 36, 1: 61-88.
Penn, Helen. 2002. The World Bank's view of early childhood. *Childhood* 9, 1: 118-132.
Peterson, V. Spike. 2003. *A critical rewriting of global political economy: Integrating reproductive, productive, and virtual economies.* London and New York: Routledge.
Pettit, Philip. 2007. Responsibility, Inc. *Ethics* 117, 1: 171-201.
Pettman, Jan Jindy. 1996. *Worlding women: A feminist international politics.* London: Allen and Unwin.
Piper, Nicola. 2003. Bridging gender, migration and governance: Theoretical possibilities in the Asian context. *Asian and Pacific Migration Journal* 12, 1-2: 21-48.
–. 2006. Gendering the politics of migration. *International Migration Review* 40, 1: 133-64.
Porter, Elizabeth. 2006. Can politics practice compassion? *Hypatia* 21, 4: 7-123.
Pratt, Geraldine. 2004. *Working feminism.* Philadelphia: Temple University Press.
Psacharopoulos, George. 1995. *Building human capital for better lives.* Washington, DC: The World Bank.
Pyle, Jean L. 2006. Globalization and the increase in transnational care work: The flip side. *Globalizations* 3, 3: 297-315.
Pyper, Wendy. 2004. Employment trends in nursing. In *Perspectives on Labour.* Statistics Canada: Catalogue No. 75-001-XE (Winter): 39-51.

Pyshchulina, Olga. 2005. An evaluation of Ukrainian legislation to counter and criminalize human trafficking. In *Human trafficking and transnational crime: Eurasian and American perspectives*, ed. S. Stoecker and L. Shelley, 115-24. London: Rowman and Littlefield.

Radin, Margaret Jane. 1996. *Contested commodities*. Cambridge, MA: Harvard University Press.

Razavi, S. 2007. *The political and social economy of care in a development context: Conceptual issues, research questions and policy options*. Geneva: UNRISD.

RCN. 2002. *Internationally recruited nurses: Good practice guidelines for health care employers and RCN negotiators*. London: Royal College of Nursing.

Reitz, Jeffrey. 2004. Canada: Immigration and nation-building in the transition to a knowledge economy. In *Controlling immigration: A global perspective*, ed. Wayne Cornelius, Takeyuki Tsuda, Philip Martin, and James Hollifield, 97-133. Stanford: Stanford University Press.

Reynolds, T. 2005. *Caribbean mothers: Identity and experience in the UK*. London: Tufnell Press.

Rhee, Ock. 2007. Childcare policy in Korea: Current status and major issues. *International Journal of Child Care and Education Policy* 1, 1: 59-72.

Rhee, Ock, Eunseol Kim, Nary Shin, and Mugyeong Moon. 2008. Developing models to integrate early childhood education and childcare in Korea. *International Journal of Child Care and Education Policy* 2, 1: 53-66.

Rhyu, Simin. 2007. Making a better future with social investment. Speech presented at New American Foundation, 26 March, Washington, DC. http://www.newamerica.net/.

RNAO (Registered Nurses' Association of Ontario). 2008. Recruitment of internationally educated nurses (IENs). Policy Brief, November, Toronto.

Robinson, Fiona. 1999. *Globalizing care: Ethics, feminist theory and international relations*. Boulder: Westview Press.

–. 2001. Exploring social relations, understanding power, and valuing care: The role of critical feminist ethics in international relations theory. In *Ethics and international relations*, ed. Hakan Seckinelgin and Hideaki Shinoda. Basingstoke: Palgrave.

–. 2006a. Beyond labour rights: The ethics of care and women's work in the global economy. *International Feminist Journal of Politics* 8, 3: 321-42.

–. 2006b. Care, gender and global social justice. *Journal of Global Ethics* 2, 1: 5-25.

–. 2006c. Methods of feminist normative theory: A political ethic of care for international relations. In *Feminist methodologies for international relations*, ed. Brooke Ackerly, Maria Stern, and Jacqui True, 221-40. Cambridge: Cambridge University Press.

–. 2008a. The importance of care in the theory and practice of human security. *International Political Theory* 4, 2: 167-88.

–. 2008b. Sex trafficking and the political economy of care: A feminist moral analysis. Paper presented at the annual meeting of the Canadian Political Science Association, 6 June, Vancouver, British Columbia.

Robinson, Mary. 2007. The value of a human rights perspective in health and foreign policy. *Bulletin of the World Health Organization* 85, 3: 241-42.

Rohatynskyj, M.A. 2003. Individual agency, the traffic in women and layered hegemonies in Ukraine. *Canadian Woman Studies* 22, 3/4: 160-65.

Rojas, Cristina. 2004. Governing through the social: Representations of poverty and global governmentality. In *Global governmentality: Governing international spaces*, ed. Wendy Larner and William Walters, 97-115. London and New York: Routledge.

Romanow Commission. 2002. *Building on values: Report of the commission on the future of health care in Canada.* Ottawa: Government of Canada Publications.

Rose, Richard. 1991a. Introduction: Lesson drawing across nations. *Journal of Public Policy* 11, 1: 1-2.

–. 1991b. What is lesson drawing? *Journal of Public Policy* 11, 1: 3-30.

Rosemberg, Fúlvia. 2006. Multilateral organizations and early childhood care and education policies for developing countries. In *Global dimensions of gender and care work*, ed. Mary K. Zimmerman, Jacquelyng Litt, and Cristine E Bose, 75-85. Stanford University: Stanford University Press.

Ruckert, Arne. 2008. Making neo-Gramscian sense of the development assistance committee: Towards an inclusive neoliberal world development order. In *The OECD and transnational governance*, ed. Rianne Mahon and Stephen McBride, 96-116. Vancouver: UBC Press.

Ruddick, Sara. 1980. Maternal Thinking. *Feminist Studies* 6: 342-67.

–. 1989. *Maternal thinking: Toward a politics of peace.* Boston: Beacon Press.

Sabatier, P., and H. Jenkins-Smith, eds. 1993. *Policy change and learning: An advocacy coalition approach.* Boulder, CO: Westview Press.

Sainsbury, Diane. 1996. *Gender, equality and welfare states.* Cambridge University: Cambridge University Press.

Sarvasy, Wendy, and Patrizia Longo. 2004. The globalization of care: Kant's world citizenship and Filipina migrant domestic workers. *International Feminist Journal of Politics* 6, 3: 392-415.

Sassen, Saskia. 2002. Women's burden: Counter-geographies of globalization and the feminization of survival. *Nordic Journal of International Law* 71, 2: 255-74.

Sawami Ryoko. 2005. Kaigo no genba ni shinpu o fukikomu gaikokujin herupa tachi [Foreign helpers who bring new winds into the site of care]. *Fujin Koron*, 7 October, 66-9.

–. 2006. Konran suru kaigo hoken no genba kara [From the sites of confused care insurance]. *Sekai*, December, 187-95.

–. 2007. Fuiripin to Nihon: Kangoshi-kigoshi ukeire o meguri miete kuru mono [The Philippines and Japan: What is appearing through the reception of nurses and care workers]. *Sekai*, July, 152-63.

Schmidt, Vivien A. 2003. How, where and when does discourse matter in small states' welfare state adjustment? *New Political Economy* 8, 1: 127-46.

Schoppa, Leonard J. 2006a. Does lower fertility threaten feminism? *Current History* 105, 689: 112-19.

–. 2006b. *Race for the exits: The unraveling of Japan's system of social protection.* Ithaca, NY: Cornell University Press.

Sen, Amartya K. 2003. The Role of Early Childhood Investment in Development. In *Escaping the poverty trap: Investing in children in Latin America*, ed. Ricardo Moran, 75-80. Washington, DC: Inter-American Development Bank.

Sevenhuijsen, Selma. 1998. *Citizenship and the ethics of care: Feminist considerations on justice, morality, and politics*. London/New York: Routledge.

–. 2000. Caring in the third way: The relation between obligation, responsibility and care in Third Way discourse. *Critical Social Policy* 20, 1: 5.

Shachar, Ayelet. 2006. The race for talent: Highly skilled migrants and competitve immigration regimes. *New York University Law Review* 81: 148-233.

–. 2008. Operation help: Counteracting sex-trafficking of women from Russia and Ukraine. PhD diss., Georgia State University.

Shapkina, Nadezda. 2008. Operation Help: Counteracting sex trafficking of women from Russia and Ukraine. Sociology Dissertations, Paper 35. http://digitalarchive.gsu.edu/.

Shimotsuke Shimbun. 2007a. Asia myakuryu 2: Kodomo ni daigaku kyoiku o [The pulsating flow in Asia 2: University education for my children]. 22 May.

–. 2007b. Asia myakuryu 3: Ganbareba mikata mo kawaru [The pulsating flow in Asia 3: Perspectives will be changed with efforts]. 23 May.

Skrobanek, Siriporn. 1998. Set me free. *New Internationalist* 305. http://www.newint.org/.

Smith, Susan J. 2005. States, markets and an ethic of care. *Political Geography* 24: 1-20.

Somers, Margaret, and Fred Block. 2005. From poverty to perversity: Ideas, markets, and institutions over 200 years of welfare debate. *American Sociological Review* 70, 2: 260-87.

Son Won-sok. 2007. Kango-kaigo bunya no gaikokujin ukeire seisaku to sono kadai [The policy for receiving foreign nurses and care workers and its issues]. In *Ibunka kan kaigo to tabunka kyosei: Dare ga kaigo o ninaunoka* [Elder care in a multicultural society: Who shoulders elder care?], ed. Chizuko Kawamura and Won-sok Son, 72-115. Tokyo: Akashi.

Spitzer, Denise, Anne Neufeld, Margaret Harrison, Miriam Stewart, and Karen Hughes. 2003. My wings have been cut, where can I fly? *Gender and Society* 17, 2: 267-86.

Spitzer, Denise, and Sara Torres. 2008. Gender-based barriers to settlement and integration for live-in-caregivers: A review of the literature, CERIS Working Paper No. 71, CERIS, Toronto.

Stasiulis, Daiva. 2008. Revisiting the permanent-temporary labour migration dichotomy. In *Governing international labour migration: Current issues, challenges, and dilemmas*, ed. Christina Gabriel and Hélène Pellerin. UK: Palgrave-Macmillan.

Stasiulis, Daiva K., and Abigail B. Bakan. 2003. *Negotiating citizenship: Migrant women in Canada and the global system*. Basingstoke, UK: Palgrave-Macmillan.

Stone, Diane. 2000. Non-governmental policy transfer: The strategies of independent policy institutes. *Governance* 13, 1: 45-70.

Sugimoto Kiyoe. 1998. Fukushi kokka to kazoku [The welfare state and the family]. *Journal of National Women's Education Centre of Japan* 2: 13-22.

Suh, Jung-hae. 2007. Vision 2030 seeks synergy effects from welfare and development. Korea Net, 5 January. http://www.korea.net/.
Sul, Kwang-Eon, Kyungsoo Choi, Hasuk Yun, Hanwook Yoo, Joonhyuk Song, and Yoon Young Cho. 2006. *Directions for social policy in changing economic and social conditions.* Seoul: Korea Development Institute.
Suzuki, Nobue. 2007. Carework and migration: Japanese perspectives on the Japan-Philippines economic partnership agreement. *Asian and Pacific Migration Journal* 16, 3: 357-81.
Takagi Hiroshi. 2006. Gaikokujin kaigo rodosha ukeire no tenbo to kadai: "Shohin" ka suru kaigo rodo [The prospects and challenges of the reception of foreign care workers: The "commodification" of care labour]. *Rissho shakai fukushi kenkyu* [Rissho social welfare study] 7, 2: 55-62.
Takeda, Hiroko. 2008. Structural reform of the family and the neoliberalisation of everyday life in Japan. *New Political Economy* 13, 2: 153-72.
Tanaka Izumi. 2007. Fuiripinjin herupa: Kaigo genba deha ko hyoka [Filipino helpers: The high evaluation at caring sites]. *Monthly kaigo hoken joho* 84: 16-18.
Tastsoglou, Evangelia, and Alexandra Dobrowolsky, eds. 2003. *Women, migration, and citizenship: making local, national, and transnational connections.* 2nd ed. Burlington, VT: Ashgate.
Tolstokorova, Alissa. 2009. Costs and benefits of labour migration for Ukrainian transnational families: Connection or consumption? *Cahiers de L'URMIS* 12. http://urmis.revues.org/.
Tronto, Joan C. 1993. *Moral boundaries: A political argument for an ethic of care.* New York: Routledge.
–. 2002. The "nanny question" in feminism. *Hypatia* 17, 2: 34-51.
–. 2005. Care as the work of citizens: A modest proposal. In *Women and citizenship,* ed. M. Friedman, 130-47. New York: Oxford University Press.
–. 2008. Is peacekeeping care work? A feminist reflection on the "responsibility to protect." In *Global feminist ethics: Feminist ethics and social theory,* ed. Rebecca Whisnaut and Peggy DesAutels, 179-200. Plymouth, UK: Rowman and Littlefield.
True, Jacqui. 2003. Mainstreaming gender in global public policy. *International Feminist Journal of Politics* 5, 3: 368-96.
Truong, Thanh-Dam. 2003. Gender, exploitative migration, and the sex industry: A European perspective. *Gender, Technology and Development* 7, 1: 31-52.
Tsutsui, Takao, and Naoko Muramatsu. 2005. Care-needs certification in the long-term care insurance system of Japan. *Journal of the American Geriatrics Society* 53, 3: 522-27.
UNDP (United Nations Development Program). 2007a. Human income and poverty. http://hdrstats.undp.org/.
–. 2007b. Trafficking in human beings in the commonwealth of independent states (CIS). Discussion Paper., September.
UNESCO (United Nations Educational, Scientific and Cultural Organization). 1990. World Declaration on Education for All and Framework for Action to Meet Basic Learning Needs. Jomtien, Thailand, 5-9 March. Paris: UNESCO.

–. 2000. *The Dakar Framework for Action Education for All: Meeting our commitments*, adopted by the World Education Forum, Dakar, Senegal, 26-28 April. Paris: UNESCO

–. 2003. Early childhood care and education reform in the Republic of Korea. Part 2: Early childhood education law. In UNESCO policy brief on early childhood, no. 16. Paris: UNESCO.

–. 2006. Republic of Korea: Early childhood care and education (ECCE) programs. Country profile prepared for the education for all global monitoring report 2007. *Strong foundations: Early childhood care and education*. Geneva, Switzerland: UNESCO International Bureau of Education.

Ungerson, Clare, and Sue Yeandle, eds. 2007. *Cash for care in developed welfare states*. Basingstoke: Palgrave.

UNICEF, OSCE, USAID, British Council. 2005. *Trafficking in Ukraine: An assessment of current responses*. Special report. Kyiv: UNICEF.

UNIFEM. 2005. *Progress of the world's women 2005: Women, work and poverty*. New York: United Nations Development Fund for Women.

United Nations. 2000. Convention against transnational organized crime, Annex II: Protocol to prevent, suppress and punish trafficking in persons, especially women and children, A/55/383 (adopted by the General Assembly, November 2000).

United Nations Development Fund for Women. 2000. *Progress of the world's women, 2000*. New York: UN Development Fund for Women.

United Nations Population Fund (UNFPA). 2006. *State of the world population 2006: A passage to hope – Women and international migration*. New York: United Nations.

US Department of State. 2010 *Trafficking in persons report*. Prepared by the Office to Monitor and Combat Trafficking in Persons, Washington, DC. http://www.state.gov/.

–. 2009. *Trafficking in persons report: Tier placements*. http://www.state.gov/.

Van den Anker, Christien. 2006. Trafficking and women's rights: Beyond the sex industry to "other industries." *Journal of Global Ethics* 2, 2: 163-82.

Van der Gaag, Jacques, and Jee-Peng Tan. 1997. *The benefits of early child development programs: An economic analysis*. Washington, DC: The World Bank.

Verloo, Mieke. 2005. Displacement and empowerment: Reflections on the concept and practice of the council of Europe approach to gender mainstreaming and gender equality. *Social Politics* 12, 3: 344-65.

Vij, Ritu. 2007. *Japanese modernity and welfare: State, civil society, and self in contemporary Japan*. New York: Palgrave Macmillan.

Vila, Larissa Josephine C. 2007. Remittances: Third world's 2nd biggest source of capital. *Business World*, 9 December 2004. http://www.ifad.org/.

Wade, Robert Hunter. 2002. The United States and the World Bank: The fight over people and ideas. *Review of Radical Political Economy* 9, 2: 215-43.

Wajima Shinobu. 2005. Kango-kaigo bumon ni okeru gaikokujin rodosha no ukeire ni tsuite: Shiyosha gawa no tachiba kara [About the reception of foreign workers in nursing and caregiving sectors: From the perspective of the employers]. *Sekai no rodo* 55, 7: 20-1.

Walker, Margaret Urban. 1989. Moral understandings: Alternative "epistemology" for feminist ethics. *Hypatia* 4, 2: 15-28.

—. 1998. *Moral understandings: A feminist study in ethics.* New York: Routledge.

—. 2006. *Moral repair: Reconstructing moral relations after wrongdoing.* New York: Cambridge University Press.

—. 2007. *Moral understandings: A feminst study in ethics.* 2nd ed. New York: Oxford University Press.

Walzer, Michael. 1983. *Spheres of justice: A defense of pluralism and equality.* New York: Basic Books.

Webb, Philippa. 2003. Legislating for care: A comparative analysis of long-term care insurance laws in Japan and Germany. *Social Science Japan Journal* 6, 1: 39-56.

Weinbaum, Batya, and Amy Bridges. 1979. The other side of the paycheck. In *Capitalist patriarchy and the case for socialist feminism*, ed. Z. Eisenstein, 190-205. New York: Monthly Review Press.

Weitzer, Ronald. 2007. The social construction of sex trafficking: Ideology and the institutionalization of a moral crusade. *Politics and Society* 35, 3: 447-75.

Werbner, Pnina. 2005. The translocation of culture: Community cohesion, and the force of multiculturalism in history. *Sociological Review* 53: 745-68.

White, Julie, and Joan Tronto. 2004. Political practices of care: Needs and rights. *Ratio Juris* 17, 4: 425-53.

Williams, F. 1989. Social policy: A critical introduction. In *Issues of race, gender and class.* Cambridge: Polity Press.

—. 1995. Race/ethnicity, gender and class in welfare states: A framework for comparative analysis. *Social Politics* 2, 1: 127-59.

—. 2001. In and beyond new labour: Towards a new political ethic of care. *Critical Social Policy* 21, 4: 467-93.

—. 2003. Contesting race and gender in the European Union: A multi-layered recognition struggle for voice and visibility. In *Recognition struggles and social movements: Contested power, identity and agency*, ed. Barbara Hobson, 121-44. Cambridge: Cambridge University Press.

—. 2007. How do we theorise the employment of migrant women in home-based care work in European welfare states? Paper presented to RC19 Conference, September, University of Florence.

—. 2009. *The making and claiming of care policies: The recognition and redistribution of care.* Geneva: UNRISD.

—. In press. Migration and care in western welfare states. In *Complexities of care: Globalisation, Europeanization and other strange words*, ed. Hanne Marlene Dahl and Anne Kovalainen. Cheltenham: Edward Elgar.

Williams, F., and A. Gavanas. 2008. The intersection of child care regimes and migration regimes: A three-country study. In *Migration and domestic work: A European perspective on a global theme*, ed. H. Lutz, 13-28. Hampshire: Ashgate Publishing.

Williams, F., C. Tobio, and A. Gavanas. 2009. Cahiers de genre (France), migration et garge des enfants a domicile en Europe: Questions de citoyennete. *Cahiers du Genre* 46: 47-76.

Winrock International. 2001. *Nationwide survey: Trafficking women as a social problem in Ukrainian society, summary findings.* Kiev, Ukraine: The Social Monitoring Centre and the Ukrainian Institute of Social Studies.

Wong, Sau-ling C. 1994. Diverted mothering: Representations of caregivers of color in the age of multiculturalism. In *Mothering: Ideology, experience, agency,* ed. E.N. Glenn, G. Chang, and L.R. Forcey, 67-91. New York: Routledge.

World Bank. 1995a. *Building Human Capital for Better Lives.* Washington, DC: The World Bank.

–. 1995b *Investing in people.* Washington, DC: The World Bank.

–. 2002. *Integrating gender into the World Bank's work.* Washington, DC: The World Bank.

Yamazaki Takashi. 2006. Kango-kaigo bunya ni okeru gaikokujin rodosha no ukeire mondai [The issues of the acceptance of foreign workers in the nursing and caregiving sectors]. *The Reference* 661: 4-24.

Yarova, O. 2006. The migration of Ukrainian women to Italy and the impact on their family in Ukraine. In *Migration process in Central and Eastern Europe: Unpacking the diversity,* ed. A. Szczepanikova, M. Canek, and J. Grill, 38-41. Prague: Multicultural Centre.

Yeates, Nicola. 2004a. A dialogue with "global care chain" analysis: Nurse migration in the Irish context. *Feminist Review* 77: 79-95.

–. 2004b. Global care chains: Critical reflections and lines of inquiry. *International Feminist Journal of Politics* 6, 3: 364-91.

–. 2005. A global political economy of care. *Social Policy and Society* 4, 2: 227-34.

–. 2008. The idea of global social policy. In *Understanding global social policy,* 1-25. London: Policy Press.

–. 2009. *Globalizing care economies and migrant workers.* Basingstoke: Palgrave-Macmillan.

Yomiuri Shimbun. 2007. Kaigo fukushishi ni jyokyu shikaku [The higher certificate for kaigo fukushishi]. 6 March. http://www.yomiuri.co.jp/.

Young, Iris Marion. 1990. *Justice and the politics of difference.* Princeton, NJ: Princeton University Press.

–. 2006. Responsiblity and global justice: A social connection model. *Social Philosophy and Policy* 23, 1: 102-30.

Young, Mary. 1995. *Investing in young children.* Washington, DC: The World Bank.

–. 2002. Ensuring a fair start for all children: The case of Brazil. In *From early child development to human development,* ed. Mary Young, 123-44. Washington, DC: The World Bank.

Zhao, J., D. Drew, and T.S. Murray. 2000. Brain Drain and Brain Gain: The migration of knowledge workers from and to Canada. *Education Quarterly Review* 6, 3. http://www.statcan.gc.ca/studies-etudes/.

Zimmerman, Mary K., Jacquelyn Litt, and Cristine E. Bose, eds. 2006. *Global dimensions of gender and carework.* Stanford University: Stanford University Press.

Zontini, E. 2004. Immigrant women in Barcelona: Coping with the consequences of transnational lives. *Journal of Ethnic and Migration Studies* 30, 6: 1113-45.

Contributors

Christina Gabriel is an associate professor in the Department of Political Science at Carleton University in Ottawa, Canada. Her research interests include gender and migration, citizenship, and regional integration. She is the co-author of *Selling Diversity: Immigration, Multiculturalism, Employment Equity and Globalization* (2002) and is the co-editor of *Governing International Labour Migration* (2008). She has contributed chapters to various edited collections, focusing on issues such as gender and migration, border control, temporary migrant workers, and North American regional integration.

Olena Hankivsky is an associate professor in the Department of Political Science, and adjunct professor in the Department of Women's Studies at Simon Fraser University. She is the author of *Social Policy and the Ethic of Care* (2005).

Rianne Mahon holds a CIGI Chair in Comparative Social Policy at the Balsillie School of International Affairs and is a professor in the Department of Political Science, Wilfrid Laurier University in Waterloo. Her earlier work focuses on unions and post-Fordist labour markets in Canada and Sweden from a gender and class perspective. Over the last decade, she has produced numerous articles and book chapters on the politics of child care, seen as part of a broader gendered process of redesigning welfare regimes. Her current work focuses on the role of international organizations in disseminating child-care and early childhood development policy discourses and the (contested) translation of such ideas in Argentina, Canada, and Mexico, at the national and subnational scales.

Hironori Onuki is a PhD candidate in political science and a Graduate Associate at the York Centre for Asian Research at York University in Toronto. He has produced articles and book chapters, focusing on issues such as global labour migration, agro-food system, and the critical theory of International Political Economy. His doctoral dissertation analyzes global labour migration and the neoliberal restructuring of global political economy in the context of Japan.

Ito Peng received a doctorate from the London School of Economics. She is a professor of sociology and public policy in the Faculty of Arts and Science, University of Toronto, and an associate researcher for UNRISD. She teaches political sociology, comparative welfare states, and public policy, specializing in family, gender, and labour market policies, and has written extensively on these topics. Her current research includes an exploration of social investment policies in Canada, Australia, Japan, and South Korea; an international comparative research project on demography, gender, and care migration; and an international comparative research project on labour market dualization.

Fiona Robinson is an associate professor of political science at Carleton University. She is the author of *Globalizing Care: Ethics, Feminist Theory and International Relations* (1999) and *Human Security and the Ethics of Care* (2011). Her research and teaching focus on ethics and feminist theory in international relations. Her work has appeared in numerous journals, including *Review of International Studies, International Feminist Journal of Politics,* and *Millennium: Journal of International Studies.*

Joan C. Tronto joined the Political Science Department, University of Minnesota, in 2009. She is also a professor emerita of political science at the City University of New York. She is the author of *Moral Boundaries: A Political Argument for an Ethic of Care* (1993), which has been translated and published in Italian and French. She is also the author of numerous book chapters and articles about the nature of care and gender. Her work has appeared in journals such as *Signs; Hypatia;* and the *American Political Science Review.*

Yuki Tsuji received a doctorate from Kyoto University, Japan, in 2011. She is an assistant professor in the College of Policy Science, Ritsumeikan University, Japan. Her research focuses on the politics of restructuring the gendered nature of the Japanese welfare state.

Fiona Williams is a professor emerita of social policy in the School of Sociology and Social Policy at the University of Leeds and a part-time professor at the Social Policy Research Centre at the University of New South Wales. She has written widely on gender and ethnicity in social policy and is currently researching the employment of migrant workers in home-based care in Europe. Her research interests focus on the place of care in contemporary society and the development of a political ethic of care. She is co-editor of *Social Politics: International Studies in Gender, State and Society.*

Index

ABC Learning, 32
abbreviations list, vii-viii
adult earners, 12, 83, 84, 181
Adversario, Patricia, 27
Africa, 28, 47
Aga Khan Foundation, 77, 90
Agathangelou, Anna, 128
agricultural workers, 52, 163, 190n11
Agustin, Laura, 130, 139, 189n5
Alberta, 52
American New Right, 92
American Sun Healthcare, 32
Amish communities, 174
Amoore, Louise, 64-65
An, Jae-Heung, 103
Antonnen, Annneli, 8, 9
Arat-Koc, Sedef, 11-12
Armstrong, Hugh, 45
Armstrong, Pat, 45
"Arusha Statement," 35
Ashbourne, 32
Asis, Maruja, 185n3
"au pair" workers, 26
Australia, 32, 42
Austria, 30

autonomy: autonomy/dependence dichotomy, 36, 181-82; disability movements, 34, 185n8; and ethics, 3, 9; gendered conceptions, 9, 131, 144; hegemonic masculinity, 130, 136-39; interdependence, 15-16, 25, 35-38, 113, 181-83, 189n4; liberalism, 112, 182; political ontology, 131; relational, 9-10, 17, 35-36, 113, 135-36

B-Dimayuga, Carmina, 68
baby boom generation, 46
Bach, Stephen, 28, 29
Bakan, Abigail B., 44, 50
Baldock, John, 8
"Baumol's disease," 184n1
Bedford, Kate, 11, 14, 138
Bell, Daniel A., 171-72
Beneria, Lourdes, 187n5
Benhabib, Seyla, 190n13
Bennett, John, 84
Bezanson, Kate, 40
Berg, Alan, 80
Bernard van Leer Foundation, 77, 90

Bezanson, Kate, 186n2
birthrate/fertility rate, 111, 120-22, 160
Black and Migrants Women's Group, 34
Block, Fred, 96
Blyth, Mark, 96
Bolivia, 91
Bose, Christine E., 41
Bosniak, Linda, 43
Boyd, Monica, 58
Brazil, 11, 91
Brennan, D., 32
Britain: care-worker recruitment, 29; child-care policies, 23; foreign-trained nurses, 41-42; global care chain, 26, 27, 29; guest worker programs, 28-29; Kalayaan organization, 34; long-term care, 31-32; National Health Service, 26, 29; nationwide care regimes, 9, 190n14; private nursery care, 32; social investment, 103, 109-10, 180
Brown, Wendy, 114
Bruckert, C., 154

Canada: critical skills shortages, 50; Commission on the Future of Health Care in Canada, 45, 185n4; global care chain, 27; Immigration Reform and Protection Act (IRPA), 50; Live-In Caregiver Program, 11, 171-72; migrant care work recruitment, 49; public expenditures as share of GDP, 45-46; women's labour force participation, 7, 127-28. *See also* immigration regimes; Internationally Educated Nurses (IENs); nurses
Canadian Charter of Rights and Freedoms, 52
Canadian Institute for Health Information, 48-49
Canadian Nurses Association (CNA), 46, 47, 50
care deficits: Africa, 28, 47; Canada, 47; crisis of care, 11, 28, 30, 41, 50, 59, 81, 158; global differences, 28, 30-31, 36; Northern hemisphere, 11, 30-31, 47; sex trafficking connection, 146, 161; socioeconomic policies, 47, 158, 160, 178
care ethics. *See* ethics of care
care-giving models, 1-17; dual earner/carers, 14, 37, 82; family-based, 62-63, 64, 95, 119, 120-22; male breadwinner, 6-7, 21, 28, 36, 82, 95, 181; migrant-in-the-family, 23; Nordic countries, 82, 83, 105; standardization, 23-24, 31-32, 63; state-supported, 8, 23, 32-33, 105, 107, 115; universal child care, 105, 107
care-giving sector, Japan: "Angel Plan"/"New Angel Plan," 116, 120; child care, 111-12, 116, 120, 188n5; discrimination experienced by caregivers, 62-63, 64, 69, 71, 72, 74; early childhood education (ECE) programs, 123-24; elder care, 62-63, 64, 69, 117-20, 123, 188nn2-3, 188n8; family-based, 62-63, 64, 119, 122, 123, 188n8; IPS Tokyo care giving Academy, 69; *kaigo fukushishi* (certified care workers), 61-63, 69-71, 186n6, 186n7; *kaigo herupa* (care helpers) level two, 69-70, 71-72, 74, 119; long-term care insurance (LTCI), 63, 70, 74, 116, 117-20, 123; migrant care workers, 60, 67-68, 73-74, 157, 186n2, 186n6; preventive approach to care (*kaigo yobō*), 118; resident training programs, 69-71, 186n9; socialization of care, 120-24. *See also* Filipino care workers; Japan
care-giving sector, Korea: child care, 97-98, 104-8, 110, 187n1; early child education and care (ECEC), 97-98, 104, 105-6; early childhood care (ECC) programs, 97-98, 101, 105; early childhood education

(ECE), 97-98, 101-3, 104-6; elder care, 94, 187n2; "Haekwons," 102, 187n4; long-term care insurance (LTCI), 94; social care expansion, 97-100, 104, 105, 107, 108-10. *See also* Korea

care provision: defamilialization, 7, 8, 9, 11, 115, 116, 188n8; definition, 151-52, 161, 189n1; distribution, 7-8, 165, 173; familialism, 114-15, 116, 119, 123-24, 180, 188n8; gendered nature, 40-41, 119, 130, 158; marginalization, 144, 159; nationwide regimes, 8-9, 158, 161; political factors, 40-41, 134, 166-71; racialized aspects, 1, 50, 124, 129-30, 143, 151; refamilialization, 11-12; responsiveness, 35, 165, 183; social constructions, 112-16, 129, 137-38; as social right, 116, 118; socialization of, 120-24; value, 135, 138, 139, 142-44. *See also* commodification of care; ethics of care

Care Work Foundation, 70, 71

care workers: job satisfaction, 70, 71; regulation/certification, 43, 56, 118; social rights, 66-68, 115; stereotypes/stigma, 15, 136, 173-74; wages, 12, 31, 124. *See also* migrant care workers

Carens, Joseph, 171, 172, 190n11
Carnegie Foundation, 81, 90
Castles, Stephen, 44
Central Europe, 8, 30
Chang, Kimberly, 137-38
Cherepakha, Kateryna, 155, 156
child care: after-school, 120; Australia, 32; child-staff ratios, 8; daycare, 79, 81, 91; deregulation, 106, 121, 188n5; European Commission Childcare Network, 83, 85; forms of, 92, 116, 188n5; gender-equal, 83-87; home-based, 8, 23, 24; neighborhood programs, 187n5;

nursery schools, 120; public responsibility, 22-24, 105, 107; quality, 85, 106; rising costs, 28; socialization, 120-22; Soviet Bloc countries, 79; state policies, 22-24, 79, 85, 97-98, 105, 107, 116; Third Way approach, 121-22; UNESCO recommendations, 77, 80, 87, 101-2. *See also* children; early child education and care

children: child poverty, 81-82, 86-87; children's rights, 80, 83-87; pre-natal care, 81, 87; raising of, 123-24, 188nn6-7; social investment, 79-80, 101-2, 180. *See also* early child education and care

Chodorow, Nancy, 3
Choi, Kyungsoo, 104
citizenship: and care provision, 158, 183; earned citizenship, 54, 58, 176; feminist ethics of care, 175-77; global citizenship, 38; hierarchal structure, 43-44, 47-48, 58, 112, 183; migrant guest workers, 29, 171-73; non-citizen status, 53; partial citizenship, 44, 64-66; and public health system, 45, 47-48; social policy, 6, 7, 12, 13, 24-25, 183

Citizenship and Immigration Canada (CIC), 49, 50, 52
class/racial stratification, 61, 69-71, 138
CNA. *See* Canadian Nurses Association
Code, Lorraine, 165, 166
Coleman, David, 87
colonialism, 28, 41
Colombia, 91
commodification of care: child care, 23, 31; ethics of care, 7-8, 63, 178-83; market values, 180-81; migrant care workers, 23, 63, 143, 151, 162, 171-73; monetization, 7-8; moral issues, 171-75; rise of in Japan, 69, 70, 73-74; socioeconomics, 23-24, 31, 63, 110, 162; standardization, 23-24, 31-32, 63

Commonwealth of Independent States (CIS), 148-51, 157-60
Conable, Barber, 88
Craig, David, 92

Da Prat, Christine, 57
Dahlberg, Gunilla, 83
Daly, Mary, 10, 112
Davies, Matt, 65
Deacon, Bob, 35, 89
Denmark, 7, 105
developing countries: care deficits, 47, 158, 161; circuits of survival, 140-41; crisis of care, 30; disability rights, 34; health professionals, 27; poverty, 21, 31; social investment, 36-37; temporary worker programs, 45. See also global care chains; migrant care workers; North/South socioeconomic divide
DiQuinzio, Patrice, 4-5
disability rights, 9, 34, 185n8
discrimination: anti-discrimination, 29; Canadian care providers, 50, 58; class/racial stratification, 29, 61, 69-71, 124, 138; elder care workers, 62-63, 64, 66-74; gender-based, 28, 121, 149-50; home-as-workplace, 29; social/citizenship rights, 66
doctors, 26, 52, 163, 190n14
domestic workers: effects on children, 174; global care chain, 128, 140, 163, 189n6; guest worker programs, 15-16, 28-29, 54-56; Live-In Caregiver Program (LCP), 54-56, 171-72; value of unpaid labour, 6-7; wages, 12, 31
Duffy, Mignon, 1-2

early child development (ECD), 80, 82, 87-91, 187n1
early child education and care (ECEC), 77-93; background, 33, 78-81, 86-87, 187n1; developmentally appropriate practices, 90; human capabilities approach, 82; in Korea, 97-98, 104, 105-6; locally based programs, 91; neighborhood programs, 187n5; poverty reduction, 87-91, 187n3; preschool education, 78-79, 91, 97; primary education, 187n3; scientific/social policy, 81-83, 90, 91; UNESCO recommendations, 101-2. See also child care; children
early childhood care (ECC), 97-100, 101, 105
early childhood education (ECE), 97-100, 101-3, 106, 123-24
Eastern Europe, 148-50, 189n5
Ecuador, 138
Education for All (EFA), 80-81, 88
Ehrenreich, Barbara, 174
elder care: discrimination experienced by caregivers, 62-63, 64, 69, 71, 72, 74; Korea, 94, 110; long-term care, 31-32, 63, 70, 74, 116, 117-20, 123; residential treatment facilities, 66; rise of care-giving sector, 186n8, 188nn2-3; rising costs, 28; socialization, 123; vouchers, 8
employment practices: deregulation, 99, 188n4; discriminatory job allocations, 70-73; forced/bonded labour, 147; forms of, 6-7, 21; full employment, 184n1; guest worker programs, 15-16, 28-29, 66, 68; parental leave, 32, 85, 92, 98, 115, 116, 120
Engster, Daniel, 151-52
Esping-Andersen, Gøsta, 6, 7, 8, 82, 83
ethics of care, 127-44; accountability, 190n15; autonomy, 9-10, 35, 38, 112, 113, 131, 135, 144; background, 2-9, 16, 35, 92, 128-29, 130-36; contextual sensitivity, 35, 133-34, 142, 152-54, 183; epistemology, 134-36, 164-65, 168; geopolitical context, 34-37, 133-34, 142, 152;

interdependence, 15-16, 25, 35-38, 113, 181-83, 189n4; moral discourses, 129-30, 164-66; profit/quality, 32, 85, 189n4; public/private, 133, 152, 158, 169, 181; relational ontology, 131, 134, 152, 163-64; responsibility, 132-33, 142-43, 152, 166-71, 189n4; right to hospitality, 172-73, 190n13; social-care discourse, 92, 113-15; women's work, 127-28, 130-36, 137, 140, 141, 142, 158. *See also* feminist ethics of care; justice; political economy of care

Eurocarers, 34

European Trade Union Confederation, 34

European Union (EU): care discourses and policies, 32-33, 92-93; choice for service use, 32; global care chains, 26-29; migrant care work recruitment, 26-29; Recommendation on Childcare (1992), 34; women in the labour force, 92; work/life reconciliation, 8-9

European Women's Lobby (EWL), 33-34

exploitation of care workers: class/racial stratification, 69-71; Filipino care workers, 64-66, 71-74; home-based care, 29, 55-56, 58, 171-72, 174; postcolonial relations, 138; sex work, 143, 147-48

family/families: care giving model, 62-63, 64, 95, 119, 120-23, 188n8; definition, 113; dual-earner, 14, 37, 82; female migration, 160; migrant-in-the-family, 23; OECD database, 84, 85; reunification policies, 30, 67-68; single parents, 84, 98, 153; transnational, 12

feminist ethics of care, 129-36, 162-77; advantages, 173-75; citizenship, 175-77; commodification of care, 162-63, 178-83; components, 163-71, 180; epistemology, 164-65; justice approach, 171-73, 183; moral criteria, 135, 140, 142, 165-66, 171-75, 188n2; ontology, 163-64; responsibility, 163, 165, 166-71, 175, 177, 183

feminization of care, 130, 158

feminization of migration, 39, 42-43

feminization of survival, 12, 15-16, 42, 140, 153, 182

Filipino care workers, 60-74; class/racial stratification, 69-71; discrimination, 66-74; as entertainers, 71-73; government role, 189n6; Licensed Filipino Caregivers Association in Japan (LFCAJ), 72; limited financial options, 66-67; linguistic-cultural barriers, 70, 72; Live-In Caregiver Program (LCP), 55-56; perception of, 67-68, 73-74; political rights, 71-73; qualification process, 61-62, 63, 69, 70, 71, 186nn6-7; socioeconomic rights, 64-71

Filipino Nurses Support Group, 56

Finland, 23

Fisher, Berenice, 165

Folbre, Nancy, 12

France, 23, 26-27

Fraser, Nancy, 10, 13, 170, 184n2

French, Peter, 190n5

Gabriel, Christina, 39-59

gender/gender equality: autonomy/dependence, 9-10, 36, 181-82; child care, 85, 122; divisions of labour, 33, 130; essentialism, 131, 136; gender mainstreaming, 35, 114, 117, 185n10; globalization, 136-39, 142, 143-44; hegemonic masculinity, 130, 136-39; interdependence, 181-82, 183; in Japan, 124, 188n1; masculine/feminine realms, 40-41; moral development

Index

differences, 3; social-care discourse, 114-15, 116, 119; social investment, 31, 79, 81, 180; social reproduction, 6-7; stereotypes, 4, 136, 181; World Bank projects, 87-88, 92. *See also* power relationships
Germany, 27, 28-29, 188n3
Gilligan, Carol, 3, 130-31
Glendinning, C., 7
global care chains: background, 1, 11-14, 22, 24, 25-29, 42-43; citizenship rights, 171-73, 175-77; family reunions, 30, 68; global South, 25-26, 44, 61, 78; health-care sector impact, 26-29; social policy, 10-14, 36, 179; socioeconomic costs, 26-29. *See also* transnationalization of care
global justice, 34-37, 136, 163, 183
global South: children's rights, 14, 87; global care chain, 25-26, 44, 61, 78; IMF policies, 178-79; inclusive liberalism, 14, 87; women's empowerment, 14; World Bank focus, 93, 179. *See also* developing countries; global care chains; North/South socioeconomic divide
globalization: definition, 2; gendered aspects, 136-39, 142, 143-44; international division of labour, 185n1; moral discourses, 129-30; national/global divide, 182-83; practice-centered perspective, 64-65; skilled migrant workers, 49
Gornick, Janet, 85
Grasswick, Heidi, 168
Greece, 23
Green, Jill, 57
Groenhout, Ruth, 189n4

Haas, E., 96
Hadley, Fran, 57
"Haekwons," 102, 187n4
Hankivsky, Olena, 5, 145-61

Hashimoto, Ryūtarō, 119-20
health-care sector: bullying, 190n14; global care chain impact, 26-29; as national symbol, 45; neoliberal restructuring, 45-46
Heckman, J.J., 82
Held, Virginia, 1, 3, 132, 134
Higuchi Keiko, 119
Himmelweit, Susan, 7
Hochschild, Arlie, 12, 42, 173
Holden, C., 31-32
home-based care: children, 8, 23, 24; elders, 119; Live-In Caregiver Program (LCP), 54-56; transnational dimensions, 25-34; workplace exploitation, 29, 55-56, 58, 171-72, 174
Honda Yuki, 123
Hooper, Charlotte, 137
Hulme, Rob, 96
human capital: capabilities, 33; Korean policy, 101-3, 105; stages, 82; World Bank investment, 78-79, 80, 88-89
Human Resources and Skills Development Canada (HRSDC), 52, 53
human rights: autonomy, 182; Filipino care workers, 74; IENs in Canada, 52; international organizations, 34, 37, 139; sex trafficking, 141; world citizenship concept, 13, 96
human security, 146
human trafficking, 145-61; background, 146-47, 157; globalization, 148-49; human rights, 141-42; International Organization for Migration, 147-48; narratives, 154-57; preventive actions, 148, 160, 161; push/pull aspects, 148-51; socioeconomics, 137, 157-60; StoptheTraffick.org, 156-57; Tier II watch countries, 148; trafficking of women, 140-41, 153; UNDP report on CIS states, 157. *See also* sex trafficking
Hypatia, 4-5

IEN. *See* Internationally Educated Nurses
ILO. *See* International Labour Organization
Im, Chae-Won, 103
immigration regimes, 49-56; criteria, 24-25, 49, 50-51, 52, 55; desired/less desired dichotomy, 48, 49; fast-track applications, 51-52; global care chains, 11-14; guest workers, 15-16, 28-29, 54-56, 171, 190nn11-12; internal stratification, 44-45; irregular migrants, 171, 190n11, 190n13; Japan, 179; landed immigrant status, 49, 50; Live-In Caregiver Program (LCP), 54-56; occupations lists, 50, 53, 55; permanent status, 50-52, 53-54, 55; provincial nominee programs (PNPs), 51-52; racism, 12; skilled workers, 40, 49, 50-51, 52, 54, 58, 185n1; subjects of rights, 13-14, 28, 29, 52; temporary migration, 52-53
indentured labour, 147
India, 27
Indonesia, 26, 60, 128
Inoguchi, Kuniko, 122
insurance systems: long-term care insurance (LTCI), 63, 70, 74, 94, 116, 117-20, 123; social insurance, 28, 37, 82-83
Inter-American Development Bank, 90
interdependence, 15-16, 25, 35-38, 113, 181-83, 189n4
International Labour Organization (ILO), 34, 37, 147
International Monetary Fund (IMF), 79, 96, 99, 110, 178-80
international organizations (IOs), 95-97, 101, 103, 110
international reproductive labour: migration patterns, 22, 24, 61; new forms, 27, 73; recruitment/training, 26-29, 49, 68; social policy, 22, 24, 26
Internationally Educated Nurses (IENs), 48-58, 185n2; Australia, 42; Canadian Experience Class (CEC), 53-54; credentialing, 51, 54, 56-59; desired/less desired migrants, 48, 49; Federal Skilled Worker category, 50-51; Live-In Caregiver Program (LCP), 54-56; percent of RN workforce, 48-49; Provincial Nominee Programs (PNPs), 51-52; source countries, 49; Temporary Foreign Worker Programs (TFWPs), 52-53
Ireland, 41
irregular migrants, 171, 190n11, 190n13
Isenman, Paul, 80
Italy, 23
Iversen, Torben, 184n1

Jackson, Andrew, 93
Japan, 60-74, 116-24; birthrate, 111, 120-22; care deficit, 62-63; coalition governance, 117, 118, 188n1; Democratic Party, 122; Economic Partnership Agreement (EPA), 60, 62; gender equality, 120, 188n1; Hashimoto administration, 119-20; immigration policy, 179; Koizumi administration, 117, 121; Korean-Japanese social inclusion, 74; Liberal Democratic Party, 117, 118, 188n1, 188n3; Ministry of Health, Labour, and Welfare (MHLW), 61, 62, 117-18, 120, 121, 186n8, 188n2, 188n5; Nihon Keidanren, 62; official development assistance (ODA), 62; parental leave, 85, 92, 98, 115, 116, 120, 188n8; patriarchal system (*ie seido*), 117; public education reforms, 188n7; rise of nation-welfare state, 63, 74, 116; social assistance system (*sochi*

seido), 116; social policy reforms, 116-20, 124; women in labour force, 63, 106, 116, 121; work/care balance, 121-22. *See also* care-giving sector, Japan; Filipino care workers; Japan-Philippines Economic Partnership Agreement
Japan Association of Corporate Executives, 120
Japan Federation of Employers' Association (NIKKEIREN), 118, 120-21
Japan International Care Aid Organization (JICAO), 69
Japan International Corporation of Welfare Services (JICWEL), 62, 63
Japan-Philippines Economic Partnership Agreement (JPEPA), 60-74; background, 61-64; economic rights, 69-71; employment opportunities, 70-71; implementation, 63-64, 73, 74; partial citizenship, 64-66; *tokutei katsudo* (designated activity) visas, 70. *See also* Filipino care workers
Japanese Trade Union Confederation (RENGO), 118, 120-21
Jeans, Mary Ellen, 57
Jenkins-Smith, H., 96
Jenson, Jane, 33
Jolly, Richard, 80
Jones, Phillip, 87
Jung, Na, 102
justice: contexts, 171-73, 183, 190nn7-8; distributive justice, 14-15, 169-70, 182-83; ethics/morality, 133, 171-73, 183; global/social justice, 33, 34-37, 90-91, 136, 163, 183, 189n5, 190n7; rule of law, 189n5, 190n7; traditional theories, 172-73, 183

Kant, Immanuel, 172-73
Kempadoo, Kamala, 151
Keynesian welfare state, 85

Kim Dae-jung, 99, 103, 109, 180
Kim, Yong-Soon, 103
Kingma, Mireille, 46
kinship ties, 37, 42
Kittay, Eva, 133
Klein, Naomi, 190n8
Kofman, E., 31, 36, 43
Koizumi, Jun'ichirō, 117, 121
Kojima, Takaki, 70
Korea, 94-110; Asian economic crisis, 97; child-care reform process, 104-8; fertility rate, 98, 100, 105, 107; government ministries, 101, 102, 103, 105-7; investment in human capital, 101-3, 105, 109; Kim Dae-jung policies, 99, 103, 109, 180; maternity leave, 98; National Basic Livelihood Security Program, 98, 99-100; OECD membership, 99, 101, 104; parental leave, 98; per capita income, 100; policy learning and transfer, 95-97, 101, 104, 109-10; political democratization, 99, 101; political economy, 100-4; presidential commissions, 100, 101-2, 106; Roh Myoo-hyun policies, 100-3, 108-9, 180; social capital, 103-4; social cohesion, 103-4; social investment, 100-4, 105, 108, 109-10; social service sector, 107-8, 109, 110; social spending as percent of GDP, 99, 100; socioeconomic transformation, 98-99; *Vision 2030*, 100, 107; women in labour force, 98-99, 103. *See also* care-giving sector, Korea
Korea Development Institute, 103
Korean Childcare Teachers' Association (KCTA), 106
Korean Private Childcare Provider's Association, 106
Korean Women's Development Institute (KWDI), 105, 106

Kuba, Yoshiko, 74
Kyzyma, I., 153

La Strada, 150, 155, 156
labour force participation by women: EU emphasis, 92; gender equality, 85-86, 92, 103, 114-15; Japan, 106, 116, 121; Korea, 98-99, 103; rising rates of, 2, 7, 79, 98, 116, 127-28, 178; work/life reconciliation, 8-9
labour market deregulation, 99
labour standards, 37
Latin America, 33
Lawson, Victoria, 16
Lee, Myung-bak, 94
Lefebvre, Henri, 65
Leitner, Sigrid, 115
Lewis, Jane, 7, 9, 112
liberalism, 92, 104, 112, 133, 137-38, 181, 184n1, 189n5
Ling, L.H.M., 137-38
Lister, Ruth, 7
Litt, Jacquelyn, 41
Little, Lisa, 47
Live-in-Caregiver Program (LCP), 11, 52, 171-72
long-term care corporations, 31-32
long-term care insurance (LTCI), 63, 70, 74, 94, 116, 117-20, 123
Longo, Patrizia, 13, 172
Lorde, Audre, 173-74
Luxton, Meg, 40, 186n2

Macklin, Audrey, 127, 141
Mahon, Rianne, 1-17, 77-93, 96, 104, 115, 151, 158, 178-83
mail-order brides, 140, 141, 189n6
Malarek, Victor, 159
Malaysia, 26
male breadwinner system, 6-7, 21, 28, 36, 82, 95, 181
Marshall, T.H., 48, 65-66, 175
masculinity discourse, 130, 136-39
maternity leave, 98

McIntosh, Mary, 6-7
McLaughlin, E., 7
McNeil-Walsh, Colleen, 41
medicare, 45, 47
Mexico, 13, 33
Meyer, John W., 96-97
migrant care workers: accountability, 190n15; care deficit in home countries, 28, 67, 179; commodification, 23, 63, 143, 151, 162, 171-73; conditional cash transfers, 10-11; direct payments, 23; family reunification, 30-31, 67-68; forms of inequality, 25, 28-29, 48, 49, 58, 67-68; licensure requirements, 56-59; Live-In Caregiver Program (LCP), 54-56; motivation, 66-68, 159, 161, 190n10; narrative accounts, 155-57; prevalence of, 11-12, 24, 128, 162, 179, 189n2; recruitment/training, 26-29, 32, 49, 69-70, 72, 179; remittances, 12, 27, 31, 67, 154, 162, 179; social movements, 33-34; socioeconomic rights, 28, 29, 52, 58, 66-68, 69-73, 172-73, 190n13. *See also* exploitation of care workers; Filipino care workers; global care chains; human trafficking
migration: definition, 146; International Organization for Migration, 147-48; motivation, 145-46, 148-51, 154-55, 156, 159, 161, 190n10; patterns, 21-29, 30, 129, 140-41, 189n2
Mill, John Stuart, 82, 173
Miller, David, 171
Mills, Charles, 168, 190n7
Moldova, 147
Molyneux, M., 11, 33
moral crusade, 139-40
moral ethnography, 135, 140, 142, 188n2
moral knowledge, 134-35
moral philosophy, 164

moral psychology, 130
morality: care provision discourses, 129; central practices, 131; expressive-collaborative theory, 164-65, 172; justice approach, 171-73, 183; sex work discourse, 139-42; stages of, 132-33. *See also* ethics of care; justice
Moss, Peter, 83
mothers: as care-work consumers, 23; global care chains, 12, 25-26, 29, 30, 153; home education, 91, 123; moral values of mothering, 3-4, 30, 173; mother-child relationship, 132-33, 173; single mothers, 98, 153; social investment policies, 33, 85, 87-89, 91, 98; state-sponsored mother-substitutes, 11, 23
Myers, Robert G., 80

nannies, 15-16, 23, 39, 128, 189n6
nation-welfare states: global interdependency, 36; governance of care labour, 43; Japan, 63, 74; Korea, 98-100, 109, 110; nursing shortages, 39, 41-42, 45-48; power relations, 44-45, 115-16; rise of, 6-7, 10, 28; social expenditures, 24, 28, 112
national security, 129
nationwide care regimes: background, 8-9, 10; cash or tax allowances, 8, 23, 32-33, 115, 119, 122; transnational aspects, 22-25, 30-31
neocolonialsim, 2
neoliberalism: care provision restructuring, 40-41, 60-61, 114, 115, 117, 143; gender equality, 121-22; in Japan, 123-24; masculinity discourse, 138-39; migrant worker assumptions, 40, 49; moral discourses, 129-30; nationwide care regimes, 9; political ethics of care, 2; social reproduction, 11-12, 64- 65, 73-74; socioeconomic policies, 78, 79, 103, 178-83
neuroscience, 81, 90, 91
New American Foundation, 100-1
New Zealand, 41
NGOs. *See* non-governmental organizations
Niemann, Michael, 65
non-governmental organizations (NGOs): human rights, 139, 148, 150, 160; social investment policy, 96, 104, 106-8; social justice, 33; transnationalization of care, 179
Nord Anglia, 32
Nordic social policy model, 82, 83
North/South socioeconomic divide: care deficits, 28, 30, 47, 59, 146, 178, 182; circuits of survival, 140-41; global justice, 37; inequalities between, 93; social reproduction labour, 44. *See also* developing countries; global South
Norway, 27
nurses: bullying, 190n14; global care chain, 26-27, 31, 43, 189n6; health-care sector restructuring, 46-47; IENs as percent of RN workforce, 48-49; nursing shortages, 39, 41-42, 45-48, 47, 48; permanent resident status, 52; regulation of registered nurses, 56-58; as skilled occupation, 54, 58; training/credentialing, 31, 41-42, 46-47, 56-59. *See also* Internationally Educated Nurses

object-relations theory, 3
O'Connor, Julia, 9
OECD. *See* Organization for Economic Cooperation and Development
Ontario, 47-48, 56-58
Onuki, Hironori, 60-74, 115
Organization for Economic Cooperation and Development

(OECD), 77-93; *Babies and Bosses,* 82, 83-86, 91-92, 121-22; compared to World Bank, 91-93; Directorate for Employment, Labour and Social Affairs (DELSA), 82, 83-87; European social policy model, 92-93; family database, 84, 85; gender pay gap, 120; geopolitical headquarters, 92-93; governance and financial reforms, 103; healthcare sector restructuring, 45; Korea joins, 99, 101; Lyon Summit (1996), 119-20; poverty reduction, 87-91; social investment policy, 2, 10-11, 33, 96, 110, 119-20, 179-80; *Starting Strong,* 33, 83, 84, 92; women's labour force participation, 7, 85-86, 92; work/life reconciliation, 8-9, 10-11, 33, 84-85. *See also* early child education and care
organized crime, 139, 140, 146-47
Orloff, Ann, 9
Ostner, Iona, 7

Parent, C., 154
parental leave, 32, 85, 92, 98, 115, 116, 120
parochialism, 170-71
Parreñas, Rhacel Salazar, 12, 22, 30, 44, 65-66
Pateman, Carole, 168
paternalism, 170-71
paternity leave, 32, 98
patriarchal societies, 2
Pattanaik, Bandana, 151
Peck, Jaime, 10-11
Peng, Ito, 94-110, 111, 115, 116
Penn, Helen, 90
Pettman, Jan, 136, 138
Philippine femininity, 66
Philippines: Association for Overseas Technical Scholarship (AOTS), 62, 64, 186n9; Canadian live-in caregiver program, 68; Economic Partnership Agreement (EPA), 60; global care chain, 12, 13, 26, 27, 41, 128, 179, 189n6; Philippines Overseas Employment Administration (PIEA), 189n6; Technical Education and Skills Development Authority (TESDA), 61; Tropical Paradise Village (TPV), 66, 72; VGB Center for Training and Development Corporation, 68. *See also* Filipino care workers; Japan-Philippines Economic Partnership Agreement (JPEPA)
Philippine Nursing Association, 27
Pikkov, Deanna, 58
Piper, Nicola, 42
Poland, 27
policy learning and transfer: International Monetary Fund (IMF), 96, 99, 110, 178-80; international organizations (IOs), 95-97, 101, 103, 110; Organization for Economic Cooperation and Development (OECD), 96, 110, 119-20, 179-80
political economy of care, 21-38; background, 22-25; political ethics of care, 34-37; transnational dimensions, 25-34
Porter, Doug, 92
Porter, Elizabeth, 134
postcolonialism, 21-29, 22, 28, 138
poverty: anti-poverty measures, 11, 31, 33-34, 81-82, 86, 87-91, 99, 160; Asian economic crisis, 99, 100, 105; child poverty, 81-82, 86-87; CIS countries, 148-51, 157-58, 160-61, 189n2; feminization of, 12, 146, 150, 189n2; lone-parent families, 84; migrant care workers, 12, 21, 28, 31, 146
power relationships: in care provision, 4, 14; distributive justice, 14-15, 169-70, 182-83; and ethics, 128; gender equality, 42, 114, 136, 141-42, 181; nation-welfare states,